TIRED YET WIRED

TIRED YET WIRED

BREAKING YOUR CHRONIC FATIGUE CYCLE

SHARON WIRANT, MA

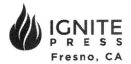

IGNITE PRESS
Fresno, CA

Copyright © 2021, Sharon Wirant

All rights reserved. No part of this book may be used or reproduced by any means, graphic, electronic, or mechanical (including any information storage retrieval system) without the express written permission from the author, except in the case of brief quotations for use in articles and reviews wherein appropriate attribution of the source is made.

Published in the United States by
Ignite Press
5070 N 6th St. #189
Fresno, CA 93710
www.IgnitePress.us

ISBN: 978-1-953655-81-3 (Amazon Print)
ISBN: 978-1-953655-82-0 (IngramSpark) PAPERBACK
ISBN: 978-1-953655-83-7 (Ebook)

For bulk purchase and for booking, contact:
Sharon Wirant Coaching
hello@sharonwirant.com
63 Emerald Street, PMB 446
Keene, NH 03431

Because of the dynamic nature of the Internet, web addresses or links contained in this book may have been changed since publication and may no longer be valid. The content of this book and all expressed opinions are those of the author and do not reflect the publisher or the publishing team. The author is solely responsible for all content included herein.

The content within this book is not intended to be a substitute for professional medical advice, diagnosis, or treatment. Always seek the advice of your physician or other qualified healthcare provider with any questions you may have regarding a medical condition.

Names of clients have been changed to provide anonymity. Their stories are shared through the authors best recollection and notes.

Library of Congress Control Number: 2021906943

Cover design by Fiaz Ahmed
Edited by Reid Maruyama
Interior design by Michelle M. White

For Rachel

Acknowledgements

More than two decades ago I planted a seed that one day I'd write a book. What that book would be about, at the time, was a mystery. The "write a book seed" germinated while I unknowingly gathered stories and interesting experiences until they were ready to sprout and bloom in the sunshine.

This book would have been a seed left wanting to grow if it wasn't for my coaches and mentors, Aimée Gianni and Molly Claire, introducing me to Everett O'Keefe from Ignited Press. Through Aimée and Molly's masterful coaching, I began to believe that not only could I heal from chronic fatigue, but also write a book. I have much gratitude and love for these two insightful and highly skilled women.

Thank you to my wonderful Book Strategist, Cathy Fyock, author of *On Your Mark: From First Word to First Draft in Six Weeks*, who kept me moving forward, opened my creative neurons with fun writing exercises, inspired my voice to come alive, and guided me along the way.

Everett O'Keefe of Ignite Press and his team of experts, Malia, Chris, and Reid, nurtured a large document file (seed) until it blossomed into a beautiful book. You and your team made this process so fun that I might have to write another book.

The powerful therapeutic coaching work with Georgina Sayce set free a big part of me that allowed the words and my work to flow. Thank you, Georgina, for being by my side on this journey.

My transformation began with Dixie St. John who started the process of stripping down layer after layer until I was finally able to find my essential self. Your intuitiveness was spot on. I am grateful for you igniting my self discovery and healing journey.

I hold much gratitude for my health care team, Dr. Ruth and Dr. Anne, for believing my story and determination in finding a solution.

My editorial team had a big job ahead of them, which they did with expediency and thoroughness. Thank you for your feedback that helped this book be born: Sandi Bixler, Cathy Fyock, Aimée Gianni, and Amanda Shyne.

There are so many within the LCS and TCC community that rallied behind me. I am thankful for Jill Wright for her wordsmithing prowess, masterful coaching, and friendship. My TCC group mates Heather, Julie, Delphia, and Tanya have been on this ride from its inception. Thank you for offering brilliant insights, heartfelt encouragement, and on-the-spot coaching that kept me writing to let my voice shine and be heard.

The biggest thank you goes to my husband, Mark, who is a true partner and always supportive no matter how nutty my idea is. This book couldn't have been written without your support and patience. I love you to the moon and back, and back again.

Contents

Introduction: What is Tired Yet Wired?   1

PART I
My Journey
BREAKING MY CHRONIC FATIGUE CYCLE

One   My Journey   7

PART II
Pulling Back the Curtain
EXPOSING THE CHRONIC FATIGUE CYCLE

Two   Factors Impacting Chronic Fatigue Recovery   27

Three   Behind the Scenes   39

Four   Why You're Still Tired Yet Wired   45

Five   The Influence of Your Behavior Habits   49

Six   The Effect of Your Thinking Habits   67

Seven   Food Habits: The Mind & Gut Connection   89

PART III

Reset + Reconnect + Recover

CULTIVATING A RESILIENT BODY, MIND, HEART, & SOUL

Eight   Tending to the Garden of You   105

Nine   Cultivating a Thriving Mindset   111

Ten   Cultivating Your Heart by Befriending Emotions   127

Eleven   Cultivating Your Soul Through Self Advocacy   149

Conclusion: The Gift of Chronic Fatigue   159

About the Author   165

Introduction

What is Tired Yet Wired?

That tired yet wired feeling is where you feel a heavy sense of sluggishness along with tiredness behind the eyes and throughout the body. Yet, despite the extreme fatigue is a feeling of being "wired" where the body is restless and the mind endlessly chatters on. Sleep is nearly non-existent, perhaps arriving in short unrestful spurts. Every day is a push to get up out of bed and fulfill obligations for the day. You push and push until either you give up because you're tired of being so tired or your body says enough is enough and shuts everything down.

There are a variety of reasons why chronic fatigue creeps into your life. You've caught a virus, been diagnosed with an autoimmune disease, or suffered from adrenal fatigue due to a highly dynamic lifestyle. Or perhaps you're simply undergoing a major change in your life, which is making you more susceptible to mental, emotional, and physical exhaustion. Today's society leans heavily on the "magic pill to fix everything" mentality. But the reality of chronic fatigue isn't so simple.

Society has conditioned us to believe that a certain way of life is the one and only way to live and be. Selling your soul to corporations, staying within the confines of someone else's definition of happiness and success instead of following your heart, keeping a full schedule that leaves little room for rest, eating processed foods to boost energy, consuming a constant barrage of visual and mental stimulation in the form of digital media and entertainment for a 24/7 experience that leaves daydreaming behind and a strong desire to compare what you do or do not have. These conditions don't encourage a thriving life or immune system; and in fact, they portray self-care as frivolous and selfish.

Stress comes in many forms that adversely affect the exquisite human nervous and immune systems. What we feed our bodies, what we think about, how we handle our emotions, and how we respond to what's happening around and within us — all of these things push our elegantly designed nervous system to work inefficiently. Humans are not simple, mechanical machines. Our bodies are complex and have a variety of factors that can exhaust the nervous system beyond its capacity, preventing us from getting into a balanced, healing state of homeostasis.

This story is about how I lost myself in a sea of noise and learned how to break my chronic fatigue cycle while healing from Lyme disease, stealth viruses, and toxic mold exposure. Hustling, overachieving, over obliging, and over helping got me in this mess, along with the genetic predisposition that responds to all the hype. The veil of brain fog, swirl of thoughts, and emotional overwhelm led me to finding my truth, aligning again with my heart by revealing and healing what I kept hidden inside. Doing this internal work rewarded me with regaining precious lost energy. How I viewed my past, present, and future created thoughts and feelings that were presumed locked in place. My past wounds and beliefs kept me stuck and unfulfilled. Eventually, my body gave up in a slow burn scenario until my fire was snuffed out. I finally became sick and tired of being sick and tired.

Persistently, like a Jack Russell Terrier scrambling down a hole toward her quarry, I looked for answers to start feeling better. Through trial and error, along with a talent for outside-the-box thinking, I applied tactics in mindset and emotional resilience practices that significantly improved my health, mental, and emotional well-being.

At the time of this writing my energy barometer is hovering at about the 95% well mark. In spite of small amounts of toxic mold still hiding and causing havoc in my body, I know exactly what to do to escort the last bits out. I nourish my body, mind, and heart, stop hiding behind chronic fatigue, heal parts of me as they are ready, provide exactly what I need when I need it with compassion, and make my opinion matter more even when someone else's opinion matters to me.

This story invites you to give yourself permission to release yourself from occupying spaces where you feel boxed in and helps you balance the scales by taking back control of who you innately are. My invitation extends to stepping into your body, aligning with your heart, and finding the courage to ignore the person elbowing your arm while whispering, "Ssshhh, you need to tuck that part of you away." Giving in, staying in your box, prioritizing others over yourself, striving for perfection to be what "they" want you to be are all huge energy leaks promoting chronic fatigue.

Within these pages I expose pieces of my inner world that most would consider unacceptable. These are parts of us that we normally hide from others, including ourselves. I share these stories and experiences for you to know that looking within is the key to healing. Shining a light on our shadows is the way out. Lastly, revealing deep parts of myself serve the purpose of reminding you that you're not the only one.

We all carry a history of experiences. While we each deal with our onslaught of thoughts and emotional discomfort differently, my intention behind this book is to propose a holistic and integrative view to reset your nervous system, reconnect with your mind and heart, and recover from chronic fatigue. Or, at the very least, be in remission longer.

The stories within are from the best of my recollection. There may be errors or slight embellishments to make the stories relevant and give a clearer visual. Any names have been omitted or changed to offer anonymity. Every person's perception of any event or circumstance is different. For me, the stories I share here are part of my truth.

Part One takes you on my journey where you'll notice how my thinking patterns, the dismissal of my emotions, and the resulting behavior sapped my body of precious energy that led to becoming vulnerable to chronic fatigue. And that my chronic fatigue cycle was set up when I was still a child.

In Part Two I pull back the curtain on chronic fatigue to give you a big picture of what's happening at the physiological level without bogging you down with technical and confusing science talk. I focus on how a maladaptive stress response is created and keeps the nervous system running in extended high alert mode. I dive into the contributing factors triggering the maladaptive stress response, explain why you're so tired yet wired, and discuss how our food choices, habitual thinking, out of balance behavioral habits, and emotional patterns keep the fatigue cycle needlessly running.

Part Three focuses on implementing a life cleanse by taking care of the garden that is you. You'll find tips and tools to create a body, mind, and emotional overhaul that brings with it renewed energy, clarity, and calmness. Your mindset and emotions, along with supporting your physical and environmental health, offers a holistic and integrative approach to help you better manage your energy to recovery.

While I am not a medical doctor, nutritionist, or psychotherapist, the tips and tools shared within are complimentary to your current medical, nutrition, and psychotherapy treatment. Life, health and therapeutic coaching helps you shift your nervous system into calmness to reduce and, in many cases, resolve chronic fatigue symptoms. Coaching does not replace medical or psychotherapy treatment. Please seek medical advice from your doctor as needed. If you experience intense emotions or are a survivor of severe trauma, please seek treatment with a qualified psychotherapy professional.

Gathering the courage to start peeling away the layers within is worth the effort and time. Awareness is the key to breaking your fatigue cycle and brings a sense of calm, freedom, and energy. Willingness and courage to look inside yourself shifts the nervous systems gears to break the chronic fatigue cycle and head to a healing state.

Gently take my hand, if you will. Come join me on a journey bound to offer relief from the grip of chronic fatigue.

PART I

My Journey

BREAKING MY CHRONIC FATIGUE CYCLE

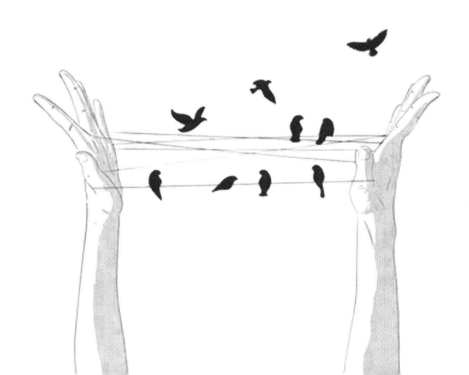

One

My Journey

Overall, I've been a healthy person with the occasional problem that medical attention easily resolved. When frequent flu-like symptoms, body aches, searing hot feet, and heavy fatigue became my normal routine, I couldn't help but think that medication would solve my illness. Periodic heavy fatigue and sleepless nights weren't uncommon throughout my life. I attributed those moments to the usual stress of a simple bad day, studying for exams, or too much on my plate. Never did I think that past experiences led to my fall with chronic fatigue, Epstein Barr virus, Lyme disease, and toxic mold illness. Little did I know that nearly all my life I was preparing for this chapter in my life.

I wish I had a spectacular story of a smoldering descent into chronic fatigue with sparks flying and smoke trailing behind. Sadly, I do not. I'm an ordinary woman who, like most everyone, had challenging life moments that left deep unnoticeable imprints. The reality is that little by little my mindset, emotions, and lifestyle gradually injected fuel that started the chronic fatigue cycle churning.

My journey doesn't begin where you might expect. It doesn't begin by landing hard in chronic fatigue and illness but while idling on the runway of my ascent. It begins as a kid curled up under a blanket reading a favorite book for the umpteenth time while nibbling on my fingernails down to the quick. As a kid, bullying caused an anxiety inside me that I didn't know how to express — to my parents, teachers, friends, and even myself. Biting my nails down to the nubs, burying my nose in books, using my imagination to make art, play with my stable of Breyer horses, and, later, real horses became my coping mechanism. I kept my voice quiet because it was easier to be seen but not heard. Eventually, suppressing my angst caused stomach pains and earaches, what we affectionately dubbed "growing pains." I'd always been in my head creating unhelpful scenarios, which made matters worse. Like Lady Gaga says, I was born that way.

Later on, as an adult struggling with an illness I wasn't even aware of, one of the first tasks my functional physician gave me, besides donating half my blood for a variety of tests, was to create a timeline of challenging life events, injuries and illnesses to find any patterns. In short, I had experienced significant challenging life events beginning with bullying, moves to new towns that required having to acclimate to new schools and friends, the removal of my wisdom teeth followed by viral infection, a significant back injury from a horse riding accident, unhealthy relationships with boyfriends and a past husband, taking a big leap at the beginning of my third decade to get a college and graduate education, all of which was followed by continuing to live a highly dynamic lifestyle with never a moment for deserved downtime.

My fatigue/trauma event timeline was eye-opening for me as my doctor pointed out commonalities. Unexpectedly getting smacked down with severe fatigue and illness appeared to come out of the blue but had actually been with me since I was a teenager. Simply succumbing to a virus that made me severely tired wasn't the full root cause of the problem. It's interesting how small traumatic or challenging life events, even with good intentions behind them, leaves an imprint in our unconscious mind and heart. Stress sends cues that set off the fight/flight response system, which impacts the chronic fatigue cycle. Putting together my own timeline of events showed a clear path of where I would end up if I didn't start taking care of me right now.

I bet you, too, will remember the catalyst for your chronic fatigue. In my junior year of high school within a week of having my wisdom teeth extracted, I likely caught mononucleosis, although was not officially diagnosed. The surgery and illness came not long after moving to a new town and reluctantly breaking up with a boyfriend from the old town. The doctor said my fatigue was nothing to worry about since I was a teenager. I often heard that I was simply "being a teenager," "fatigue was a figment of my imagination," or that I'm just one of "those" people who are always tired. Hearing those words frequently enough, you end up pushing through the fatigue, which I did, because if they thought I wasn't tired then I must not truly be fatigued.

We all have challenging moments in our lives. Mine has been no exception. These moments are part of the human experience, but we aren't taught how to take care of ourselves during these circumstances. These challenging moments are often caused by the loss of a loved one, a devastating breakup or divorce, bullying at school or at work, relocating to a new city, unexpected accidents or illnesses, caretaking for a loved one, or witnessing unfair treatment of a person or animal. Because they're "small" stressful events, we're either told or think we can "just get over it" when the body and brain need to process the emotions to then return back to the safety zone. We tend to push emotions aside either because they're uncomfortable or because society tells us they're unacceptable.

As I stepped aside to analyze how I became sick and utterly exhausted, certain patterns emerged throughout my written timeline. Always a curious, easy-going, observant kind of person, I followed the flow. Appeasing others by becoming a peacemaker helped me to avoid conflict and rejection, even though the conflict rumbled in the background inside me. That easy-going, "don't rock the boat" person had a rebellious side, too. My rebellious side isn't the kind that's angry or wants to cause harm in any way. I'm a heart-centered rebel and an outside-the-box thinker who has a hard time staying within the lines. I like paving my own path, my way. I grew up believing I could do anything as long as I had a mind for it so I saw, and still see, that I can do and be anything I want.

What I didn't know then was that my heart-centered rebelliousness needed intentionality behind it to keep me balanced. Living unintentionally meant that I didn't think or plan ahead, said yes when I really wanted to say no, prioritized everyone and everything else above myself, avoided conflict and rejection by not standing up for myself, and tried hard to control the outside noise around me by obliging anyone who needed something from me.

Living unintentionally led to a first marriage at the tender age of 19 shrouded in gaslighting and abandonment. The unpredictability of this unhealthy marriage created high anxiety that later manifested into panic attacks and Intestinal Bowel Syndrome (IBS).

While in high school my mother and I had an afterschool ritual of sharing snacks while watching *The Oprah Winfrey Show*. We enjoyed sharing snacks of frozen raspberry Zingers or butterscotch Tastykakes while watching the end of *The Guiding Light* and *The Oprah Winfrey Show* while catching up on the school day. I continued this tradition when I moved away from home whenever I could. Arriving home from work early one day, I sat down to watch *The Oprah Winfrey Show*. How serendipitous that the particular episode I was watching was about domestic violence? The list of red flags awakened what I felt deep inside. The time to leave this terribly unhealthy marriage behind was now. For the first time in my life, I made a plan.

Asking for help never came easily for me. I contrived a solution to fund my great escape by creating a side hustle that quickly took off. Not too long before recognizing that I needed to make a major change, I completed an equine sports massage certification course. My local equine community opened their barn doors for me to massage their hardworking horses. Every cent I made from my side gig was stashed and hidden in a purple velvet Crown Royal whiskey bag until the moment I could take flight.

Massaging performance horses and dogs, then later becoming a licensed massage therapist for people helped me build a self-supportive foundation and a habit of hustling and staying overbusy. I hustled from barn to barn when I wasn't working my part-time job or going to massage school, developing a habit of eating fast food meals behind the wheel of a car. This pattern of busy-ness continued while I went from town to town to collect data for both my undergraduate and later graduate research. My road warrior lifestyle was born.

Those stomach pains I experienced as a child had morphed into Irritable Bowel Syndrome (IBS). Those pesky IBS symptoms began as my first marriage deteriorated then took a brief pause as I started a new chapter in my life. IBS and an interesting migraine pattern emerged full force as I pushed myself to complete my undergraduate and then graduate degree within the shortest time frame possible. Maintaining a suppressed state of stress added a bit more fuel to start churning my chronic fatigue cycle.

It was a crisp, bright September morning as I sat in Cell Biology class listening to the instructor when suddenly the floor snapped upward like an untethered window shade opening up to let the bright sunlight in. Then everything went black while my face planted into the desktop. A raging migraine followed for a week. Doctors had no clue what was going on or how to diagnose this strange episode and thought I just fainted. The next time this interesting blackout happened, I was walking from the rental car drop-off to the ticket counter at the Eugene, Oregon airport after judging a dog agility trial over the weekend. That time I fell flat on the concrete floor. Several minutes went by before someone came up to me to ask if I was alright. Even though I felt disoriented, I eased myself up, told the Good Samaritan I was okay, then found a payphone to call for advice from my current husband. Hunkered against the plane window, a severe migraine was making itself known as I flew from the West to the East coast. After many tests, MRI's and brain scans, my neurologist suspected basilar migraines. Basilar migraines occur with the fluctuation of blood pressure. The side effects of anxiety were beginning to show. Lucky for me, my migraines went away with a significant diet change and the work I describe within these pages.

Being a quiet, more cerebral type of person, along with my easy-going rebellious self, isn't an easy combination. I'm a great observer yet a sponge of all the emotions and energy going on inside and around me. I question, analyze, and make up stories inside my head. Those ingredients simmer in the brain and body wasting precious energy setting up the perfect scenario for physical and emotional collapse.

My tendency to keep moving and working helped me build a successful massage therapy practice, start college as a 30-year-old, and build an amazing career in animal welfare. Here's where the rebel in me got me into a spot of trouble. A high school guidance counselor once told me that I wouldn't succeed in science and the business administration track was my best option. Studying massage therapy taught me that I can indeed learn science. Anatomy and Physiology was one of my favorite subjects. My Inner Rebel told me, "We're studying Biology and we'll prove my high school guidance counselor wrong!" The problem with this is that I focused on proving someone else (whose name I don't even remember) wrong when the person I needed to prove my intelligence to was myself. Proving someone else wrong drove me to overfill my plate, harshly judge my work, and achieve hard things to prove my worthiness.

I fell in love with psychology, behavior, and neuroscience. The list of classes was like a smorgasbord for me. Yes, I'll have one of everything, please! Can we say "overachiever" here? I filled each semester with at least 18 credits, if not 21. Being a biology major meant that you take classes in the morning and then labs in the afternoon. Admittedly, I was quite envious of my friends who had more space between classes as I pushed myself to the absolute limit.

The number of intense courses I took meant I simply didn't have the time to focus as deeply as I wanted and needed. I ran myself ragged between studying for my classes, collecting and analyzing data for my research projects, competing in dog sporting events, and spending time with my husband. I burnt the candle on four ends, not just two.

It's interesting that I know when I'm running on energy vapors. Weird stuff starts happening when my fuel tank is nearly on E. I remember one time when I was feeling overwhelmed and anxious because I had a major paper due, a neurophysiology exam the following day, and I had just received word to collect data from a research subject 100 miles away. I had barely been home from the last data collection trip and feeling tired. Getting into my SUV for my 50-mile ride to class, I started the vehicle, promptly shifted the gear into reverse, and hit the gas. Quickly and blindly backing up I suddenly heard a crash and rip sound. Backing out of the garage without opening the door, I ripped off the roof rack while driving through the garage door.

And then the panic attacks started rolling in. While my ex-husband was out on the town until the wee hours of the morning, panic attacks would hit me around the 2 or 3 o'clock hour. One time, out of what seemed like nowhere, a panic attack rose up in the middle of a history class in college. Frantically, I scooped up my notebook, stuffed it into my backpack, then ran out the room. I ran until that panicky feeling started to settle down. Now I know that something in the environment, a thought, or a familiar emotion caused my panic attacks. Panic attacks are due to an overload of anxiety. Anxiety is a buildup of untended emotions. Eventually, the attacks simmered down after my first marriage dissolved. Today, panic attacks are now long gone. Exploring my emotions underneath the anxiety and applying self-care practices in part three of this book has dissolved my panic attacks and anxiety.

The nonstop nature of running to school, studying, frequent week-long data collection trips, having a home life, and competing in dog agility caused a tired yet wired feeling inside my body, digestive issues and panic attacks, and started the cycle that saps my body of energy. I was spent and exhausted after graduating college with undergraduate degrees in Biological Science and Neuroscience. The sudden stop of activity left me feeling like a zombie. Sleep was difficult and unrefreshing as it's always been. I'd slowly putter around the house trying to appear like I was actually accomplishing something when I could have been taking care of myself.

Graduate school was again a fast-paced grind that fueled my habit of busy-ness and achieving. Classes, studying, assisting with labs, collecting data, researching, writing, and driving all over New England for data collection and dog competition events kept me in motion. If you can't tell by now, sitting still wasn't my style. Sitting still meant I had to feel my doubt and insecurities while my Inner Critic barked orders inside my head.

At the end of graduate school, I was again terribly drained of energy from pushing through to get everything done. My fuel tank was empty. Sleep wasn't restful, my body felt heavy, and my movement felt sloth-like. Brain fog, along with a veil of fatigue, enveloped my head. Fortunately, I didn't have any work lined up yet. This allowed me time to rest the best way I knew how and push myself to find a job in the research or animal welfare field. Even though I rested and fervently searched for work, fatigue followed me like a shadow.

The world of animal welfare was perfect for a person like me who was always ready to go. I wanted to help animals heal physically and psychologically, feel part of important work, and use my hard-earned knowledge and experience. The thing is that I brought along my habitual way of living into my professional life. We like to think our personal and professional lives are separate. They are not. They blend together whether or not we like it. And the results can be either beautiful or disastrous depending on how we navigate those boundaries.

Somehow along the way I began to lose my sense of self. I don't think it's uncommon for us to figure out the easiest route is to follow the group rather than our heart's desire. As brash youngsters it's easier to confidently dive into new opportunities. Growing older, we become more conservative and easily succumb to societal norms because it's easier. At about middle-age or our second half of life we begin to question what matters most. For me, stepping out of an academic environment that celebrated female intellect and leadership and into the real world molded by containment-type beliefs was a hard pill to swallow. At some point, my Inner Rebel submitted to the cause by taking a long slumber hidden in a faraway cubby inside me while I attended to what others expected of me until she got tired of the B.S. and began waking up.

Can you identify where you lost the true sense of who you are? Have you unknowingly silenced your Inner Rebel, too? Our Inner Rebel is our inner wisdom speaking up about what's true for us. Some call this our Inner Wisdom but I like Inner Rebel better. She's the one telling you to walk your own path, to resist conforming, and to embrace your quirkiness.

Another decade went by before I realized how I unconsciously conformed to what society expects. I found myself in crisis-oriented and highly dynamic positions in the animal welfare industry. Animal rescue is fast-paced, dynamic, and last minute. It's the nature of the business. Saving animals and helping people made my heart sing and fit my pattern of always doing, caring, and helping.

A good portion of my professional life involved working on the front lines of animal rescue. I've had the opportunity to work on crime scenes along with the F.B.I. and local law enforcement. Dog fighting raids commonly included crimes, such as drugs, weapons, gambling, prostitution, domestic violence, and animal cruelty, committed by the dog fighter defendants. Standing next to a team of women and men dressed in their S.W.A.T. assault protection gear is awe-inspiring. They ooze unshakeable confidence and fierce intimidation. You feel part of something very big and important. It's a piece of the work that's hard to let go of and walk away.

Being part of such important work became a strong magnet for me to keep on going. Playing a role alongside law enforcement to clean up the mess left behind by greedy dog fighters, overcrowded puppy mills where dogs are property for profit by the number of puppies they pump out, and mentally impaired people who hoard animals while living in squalor with misdirected love and intentions is not work for everyone, but I needed to be part of it. The bad guys are punished and those suffering mentally get the help they need. A majority of the animals get successfully rehabilitated enough to find happy and healthier homes when the case finally closes. Taking part in such a heroic line of work added to the attraction of always wanting to be part of the scene.

The fear of missing out is a magnetic pull that easily kept me in constant crisis mode and believing the necessity of always having a presence whether on the road or supervising from afar. I remember assisting with several back-to-back animal removals while taking on rotating shifts at a temporary shelter. There seemed to be a steady flow of animals needing rescue and rehabilitation. There was never much downtime to be had in between those trips. Even though I could have insisted on a break, the pull to add my name to the participant list, the fear of being viewed as difficult or weak, and the risk of losing my job were stronger. You do whatever you must to stay in the game, especially when the work is exciting and addictive. The thing is that no matter what there will always be a crisis and a strong need to help. Wanting to always be available, to be a part of the team, and to contribute my value was the perfect combination that built self-imposed pressure when what I really needed was a break.

What's not a surprise is that the way I handled my professional life was the same way I handled my personal life. I didn't want to miss out on any dog agility training or competition opportunity, social events with friends, or visiting family who live far away. The way I lived and what I gave priority to made me miss my grandmother's 90th birthday party. More heartbreakingly, because I prioritized travel, I nearly missed saying goodbye to my beloved 17 year old Jack Russell Terrier, Darla. How my heart sank when my husband greeted me upon my return with Darla barely alive on top of the coziest pillow that could be found. I'm so grateful that my Darlin' Darla waited for me to come home to say goodbye.

Clearly, my unhelpful thinking habits, dismissing how I felt and how I responded to every circumstance showed up over and over again in both my professional and personal life. The topic may be different yet my response pattern was the same. I was addicted to adrenaline. Adrenaline covered the discontent and insecurity simmering underneath until it no longer did. Running on adrenaline is a fear response that's supposed to be short-lived. It's not sustainable in the long run.

The thing about adrenaline is that it's meant for short-term activation. Our culture today is addicted to adrenaline, stimulation, and instant gratification. The human (or any species for that matter) aren't meant to run on adrenaline for hours, days, weeks, or months. The human body will break down with illness and disease from overworking. I learned this the hard way.

Mental and emotional exhaustion in a highly dynamic, compassionate, and caregiving environment comes at a heavy price and is common in any caregiving industry. It's not uncommon for an animal caregiver to give priority to the animals first, to obsessively think about the animals, and to become emotionally attached to an animal's outcome. These are a few red flags indicating compassion fatigue. These traits are mentally, physically, and emotionally draining and lead to burnout and contribute to chronic fatigue illnesses.

Unlike most caregiving roles, the animal welfare industry has the added weight of ending the life of an animal who is a public safety risk yet otherwise healthy. Having made life decisions for animals, I'd been stalked, screamed at, and had my experience and education belittled because I told the truth. There are some dogs that are a public safety risk due to their harmful behavior. The truth needed to be told to families surrendering pets to the shelter, staff who fell in love with animals they cared for a long time, a family needing to make a life-or-death decision, or a person making wrong and harmful choices to those around them. Once, as a new manager and behaviorist, I made the recommendation to euthanize an adult dog that had been surrendered because their owners couldn't take them to their new residence. Moving is one of the top reasons for pet relinquishment to animal shelters. Since the previous owners gave a sparse behavioral history on the dog, the euthanasia decision was based on the dog's aggressive behavior toward the animal caregivers in the shelter. The dog cornered a caregiver while snarling and lunging. The dog also charged and badly bit a caregiver when attempting to take him to the medical office for an exam. The behavior and bite were simply facts driving a decision that the dog was a public safety risk. Harassment and stalking by the former owners and friends began after hearing the news. Situations like these are flashbacks to those old bullying days.

There are many aspects of my professional life that felt like home but I gave too much of myself from an empty well of energy. By solely focusing on my profession rather than blending both my work and life, I created an imbalance that left me believing I was wrong about my purpose. An avid researcher and book reader, I searched for books to help me get out of my funk. One day I was rummaging in our local bookstore when Dr. Martha Beck's book *Finding Your Way in a Wild New World* literally leapt into my hands. The book resonated with me so much that I checked out her online offerings and attended a few free training sessions, eventually graduating from Dr. Beck's Life Coach Training program.

Dr. Beck talks about Wayfinder illness, which is when you get sick from not processing emotions, wild thinking patterns, and not following your internal compass. You become susceptible to viruses, bacteria, or toxins in your system. We all have an inner compass that guides us. It's why I love horses and dogs while you prefer children, cats, or no animals at all. Veering off your path, letting your thinking run wild, and ignoring emotions will send you off-kilter and will spark the chronic fatigue cycle.

Speaking of our internal compass, mine began telling me to stop running a fast-paced life. I knew something was wrong as frightening dreams, body pain, and flu-like symptoms hit me like clockwork. Whole body stiffness, aches, searing hot feet and amplified back pain, headaches, low grade fever, and fatigue washed through my body, all of which seemed correlated with travel and stressful events. Traveling for business or pleasure didn't matter. Crashing with flu-like symptoms and heavy fatigue became routine while doctors couldn't find anything wrong.

Finally, I gave in because deep down I knew I needed rest. My body was screaming to stop. My body had been sending messages that I ignored. It took a serendipitous yoga session for me to actually listen. Yoga became a calm, peaceful sanctuary for me; a peaceful retreat leaving everything outside the door. Yoga invited me to connect with my body to feel and listen to its rhythm and song. There were classes where fatigue overwhelmed me to the point where all I could do was rest in child pose the entire class. During the serendipitous session a "voice" shouted at me, loud and clear. The theme for our yoga session that day was resistance. The instructor shared bits of wisdom as she gently moved us from pose to pose. Easing into a downward dog she said, "Ask yourself what you're resisting." I swear with my life that a voice out of nowhere shouted, "Stop!" so audibly I thought everyone in the room could hear. Finally, I heard the message my body was sending me. I stopped. I resigned from the work I enjoyed because I knew I couldn't meet the expectations anymore. I cut back on social and competitive dog agility events and focused on my physical, mental, and emotional health with a new health team, therapy, and an impactful group of life and therapeutic coaches.

Before life coach training, I would come home from my work travels and, literally, crash on the sofa until I had to pack up to leave again. Exhaustion led to scrolling through emails but not responding to them, mindlessly reading social media posts, and answering texts while in my mind I was chastising myself for not getting more done and numbing out the discomfort inside my heart. I'd even mustered up the energy to attend dog training workshops and competitions, but even then several days if not weeks were needed to somewhat recover. Being hard on myself for not keeping up fueled the chronic fatigue fire even more.

While I was pondering my purpose and direction, I used the life and health coaching tools I learned, and worked one-on-one with coaches to go deep within to find answers.

By this point, I had stepped away from my career, set out to heal myself, and figure out my next chapter. Despite three months of rest and low-key activity, flu-like symptoms continued to plague me. On the good spectrum, my handy research skills found a Naturopathic doctor who specializes in fatigue. Our first task was to run bloodwork to test for hormone levels, potential viral load, measure my cortisol levels, and establish a baseline with a CBC. Twenty-something vials of blood later, my test results indicated I had reactivated mononucleosis, a few stealth coinfections, and adrenal fatigue. My hormones and thyroid were teetering on the edge, about to glide downward. We began treatment, I started feeling better, but flare-ups periodically slammed me back down. Showing up for a follow-up appointment during a flare-up, my doctor decided to pull a tick panel to test for Lyme or other tick borne disease. The test confirmed I also had Lyme disease and I was referred to a Lyme-literate doctor.

Sitting across my doctor's desk going over test findings, her assistant delivered one more test result. My doctor briefly looked at the piece of paper then with a quick flick of the wrist flipped the paper upside down. Right then I knew we had an answer. In spite of being on appropriate treatment for my current load of viruses, co-infections, and bacteria, I wasn't getting better because of an overload of toxic black mold, Ochratoxin A and Mycophenolic Acid. Mycophenolic Acid suppresses the immune system and is used to make immunosuppressant drugs for organ transplant recipients.

I hired a certified mold inspector because we needed to ensure our home was environmentally safe. To our shock and dismay, the inspector discovered toxic mold in our basement and in the entry of my studio. We had a water valve break about four months prior. The mold inspector couldn't say for sure when the mold took up residence, and so it was unclear to me if I had picked it up at home or a past work site. What we positively know is mold was found, was in my body, and my immune system was broken as a result.

Not only does mold invade your cells preventing them from doing their job, but it also takes over your brain. Mold is like a heavy, dark grey veil that drapes over your brain. I feel this drape down over my eyes, too. I swear mold has a way of twisting your thoughts into ones that are scathing insults and self-pity. The sharp jabs of insults bring up a variety of emotions that boil and bubble throughout your body. Since I couldn't drink alcohol to numb those sensations, I ended up watching *The Great British Bake Off* one after the other while patiently waiting for the calm tide to roll in.

Fortunately for me, my thoughts didn't send me off the edge. I quietly sat back and observed them but didn't attach to any of them. I'm grateful for Byon Katie's *The Work* and my coach training with Dr. Martha Beck of the *MBI Life Coach Training* program and Brooke Castillo of *The Life Coach School*. These two modalities are based on Cognitive Behavioral Therapy and the ancient theory that what we think we create and that we are not our thoughts.

I had a lot of unhelpful and interesting thoughts but employing thought work (examining thoughts to select helpful ones or create new intentional thoughts) and meditation into my daily routine stopped the swirling and overwhelming unhelpful thoughts I'd been having for years. We don't have to be our thoughts, my friends. Really, we don't.

Managing my mind while detoxing my body made a world of difference. Yet, a mask of fatigue seemed determined to hold on. Emotions started to speak up asking for help. Mind management led the way back into my body, though for me I needed to start with my body first. We're all different. Some folks do best focusing on their mindset while others from the heart. Alex Howard and his team at the *Optimum Health Clinic* helped me dig into and heal my tired and hurt emotional heart.

Being a quiet, thoughtful person who feels everything, I needed to learn the language of my body. What's it saying? What does my body need now? Before I wasn't listening to my emotions and creating unhelpful thoughts that led me to feeling more anxiety, depression, frustration, pity, and anger. Once I started stepping into my body, feeling, and being curious about what I was feeling, processing and digesting my emotions, my sleep and mood improved tremendously.

I could easily blame my pursuit of education, my past employers, my loved ones, and my house for all my ills. Life is part amazing and part sucky. We'll always have wonderful employers and awful ones, loved ones who honestly did their best and ones intent on hurting others, and stuff that happens because it just does. There's no point in staying in victim mentality mode unless you truly enjoy that pity party for one. We have one life to live, as far as I know. I don't believe we're here to purposely suffer. Life has its ups and downs; life is not linear.

As Maya Angelou says, *"When you know better, you do better."* This quote and Ms. Angelou's writings, among many others, contributed to shifting my own perception of the world and the people in my life differently. The truth is that most people are doing the best they know how. Some people decide to stay where they are while others choose to do better next time.

How I became ill is more than exposure to a virus or toxic mold. A culmination of overachieving, perfectionism, pleasing and helping others without regard to my needs and wants, and dismissing the feelings of anxiety, rejection, and anger weakened my immune system and depleted my energy. I had poorly executed boundaries, miscommunicated my needs, numbed myself through busy-ness, and showed up for others before myself, all to prove I was enough. What a toxic combination!

What are the ingredients that create chronic fatigue? A few of the ingredients are overworking, not honoring boundaries, the wrong physical or social environment, mental fatigue, emotional fatigue, and compassion fatigue. These external and internal disturbances in our lives create noise that depletes energy by signaling to the nervous system that there is a significant threat. Being in a constant state of threat weakens the immune system, making you vulnerable to illness until the energy leaks are repaired.

The way out isn't easy, that's for sure, but it is worth the freedom found by embracing your sovereignty and learning how to manage all your energy leaks. I always said I must be dependent on myself and no one else but not for the right reasons. Essentially, I gave away my power, my sovereignty. I now think "I'm here for me," instead of having to depend on myself. "I'm here for me" feels compassionate to me, like I've taken back my power and have my own back. I've reclaimed my sovereignty.

Inner work is a secret ingredient to regaining your energy. Doing the inner work of paying attention to and listening to my thought habits and emotions opened up space for me to reconnect with my Inner Rebel (or Wisdom, if you prefer). Reconnecting with my Inner Rebel ignited healing from my overload of viruses, Lyme, and toxic mold by sending my nervous system into a calm, healing state. Connecting with myself allowed me to clean up my body, mind, heart, and soul. I've embraced every emotion and their sensations in my body as they rise to the surface. I've continued to learn more about me, my needs and wants, which, in turn, stops the stress causing the nervous system to overwork. When I'm in a calm, healing state I'm able to overfill my cup of energy so I'm able to give from the extra that has spilled into the saucer instead of pushing myself to give from the few drops at the bottom of the cup. Becoming intentional in thinking habits and caring for any emotional wounds preserves and refills your energy stores. Chronic fatigue is about learning how to conserve your energy. Just like fossil fuels, our energy is a valuable commodity to be used wisely.

In the following pages I present to you a Life Cleanse process that significantly reduces or resolves chronic fatigue symptoms with an integrative and holistic approach that I've used in my own chronic fatigue healing journey. The human body depends on all parts of itself to function and heal; not one single ingredient or pill fixes it all. The healing from chronic fatigue journey is about taking care of your body, mind, heart, and overall being, your soul. It's a journey I gently guide my clients on to locate, repair, restore, and refill their energy input and output.

PART II

Pulling Back the Curtain

EXPOSING THE CHRONIC FATIGUE CYCLE

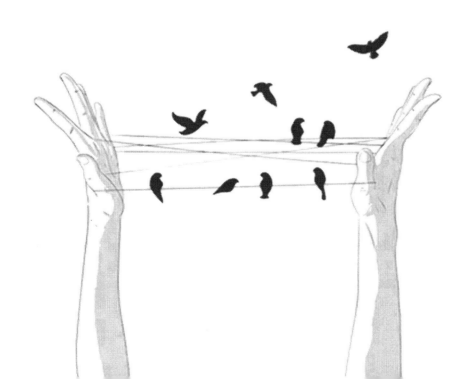

Two

Factors Impacting Chronic Fatigue Recovery

Before venturing into a therapeutic approach of processing my deeper emotional layers, I was several years into an energy producing diet, along with a mindset and positive psychology practice prior to my chronic fatigue crash. The realization hit me that additional inner work needed to be done as I sat in a circle with a few close friends on the green artificial turf inside a soccer arena watching the competitors in a dog agility competition as I felt the crash moving in.

As I was sitting with friends the feeling of absolute exhaustion gripped my entire body. How can it be, I wondered out loud, that I'm so bloody tired even though I'm on proper treatment? How can it be that I feel like a bus ran over me not once, but multiple times? The full body stiffness, low back pain, heaviness of fatigue, brightness of the lights, loud cheering from the enthusiastic crowd was making me retreat and hide as my symptoms worsened. This moment indicated to me that there are more factors to the chronic fatigue healing process.

Fatigue can persist even if you're on appropriate medication. Although viruses, challenging life moments, and chronic stress are often pinpointed as causing chronic fatigue, several additional factors can impact recovery such as your genetic tendencies in your physical body, the environment around you, and your thinking, emotional, and behavioral habits. You may carry a gene that causes an autoimmune disease, unknowingly live or work in a water damaged building, engage in toxic relationships, become mentally and emotionally fatigued from out of control thought patterns, or be simply avoiding uncomfortable feelings. These tendencies are big energy depleters that contribute toward the tired yet wired feeling and the crashes associated with chronic fatigue.

What we do know is that chronic fatigue often shows up after a challenging life event or sudden illness. Challenging life events include moments, such as completion of final exams, a difficult divorce or breakup, death of a loved one, an accident, or a stressful work or home life. With chronic fatigue there are times the fatigue is so severe that getting out of bed is near impossible, if not impossible. Sleep is not at all refreshing, no matter how many hours you rest. Flu-like symptoms return, especially after physical or mental activity, or an emotional upset. Work, plans, and fun events get put on hold indefinitely. And worry seeps in that another crash is around the corner waiting to take you back down.

The sicker I became the more I wanted to withdraw and isolate from others. The idea of having to socialize with friends or co-workers, travel for business or pleasure, show up appearing eager for meetings, or step to the start line with my dog by my side became a stressor because I knew a crash wasn't far behind. It didn't matter where I was traveling to or from; I'd dread getting into the car. Simply driving into town for groceries was exhausting. The desire to withdraw and isolate myself affected my mood and how I responded to the people around me. One time I was so tired at a competition that I often hid until my turn to run. The struggle to maintain a happy and outgoing attitude became a chore with many of the activities I enjoyed.

Through the extraction and dissecting of sources about chronic fatigue and mold toxicity, I noticed a pattern of factors impacting recovery from chronic fatigue. I derived the four factors affecting healing from chronic fatigue from the works of Alex Howard of the *Optimum Health Clinic*; Dr. Ritchie Shoemaker, author of *Surviving Mold: Life in The Era of Dangerous* Buildings; and Dr. Neil Nathan, author of *Toxic: Heal Your Body from Mold Toxicity, Lyme Disease, Multiple Chemical Sensitivities, and Chronic Environmental Illness.* The four factors that stood out include: 1) physical body, 2) environmental exposure, 3) mindset, and 4) emotional resilience (Figure 1). All four factors can be separately examined yet are intimately entwined. It may be a shock to see the words mindset and emotional resilience as factors, but they play a vital role in our well-being. Let me explain further.

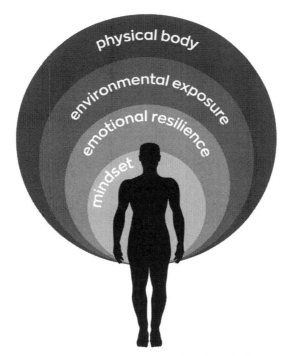

Figure 1: The Four Factors Impacting Chronic Fatigue

PHYSICAL BODY

Nature and nurture impact physical health. You may have a genetic tendency toward a specific illness, such as rheumatoid arthritis or lupus. Perhaps you're lucky not to have a genetic disposition but caught a viral illness or bacterial infection, such as Lyme disease, or were exposed to toxic mold. Viruses, bacteria, and molds are plentiful in nature. They serve a role in our environment, but our bodies may have become weakened and more susceptible to these threats.

The human body is elegantly designed to take care of microbial invaders, including viruses, bacteria, mold, inflammation, and infections. At times you need assistance from the medical community to reduce an overload of the toxins. Perhaps you have *Candida*, which is an overgrowth of the fungus *Candida albicans* in the gut, which often causes skin rashes, athlete's foot, nail or vaginal infections, brain fog, digestion issues, or autoimmune diseases. However, it can also affect memory and focus, and contribute to irritability, anxiety, and depression. *Candida albicans* typically lives in your mouth and intestines to aid digestion and nutrient absorption but causes problems when your gut's microbiome becomes unbalanced due to a high carb, sugary diet, or chronic stress. Antifungals, in addition to diet changes, are an important step to knocking back the *Candida* overgrowth to get your microbiome back into balance.

The nurture part of physical health is how you take care of yourself. The important components are what you choose to fuel and nurture your body with, including how you talk and support yourself. Fresh foods support your body all the way down to the cellular level. Fast and processed foods are manufactured to give your brain a pleasurable dopamine hit with little to no nutritional value. Unfortunately, Starbucks and McDonald's don't offer our bodies with much nutritional value. There are many different food lifestyles that support specific autoimmune, chronic fatigue, and mold toxicity illnesses. Taking care of your body down at the cellular level matters in breaking the chronic fatigue cycle.

If you're exercising regularly, eating a nutrient dense diet, and doing your inner work, yet still feeling fatigued then speak with a physician to rule out potential genetic, viral or bacterial infections, and mold toxicity.

ENVIRONMENTAL EXPOSURE

In my professional experience, the typical animal hoarding rescue scene affects the health of both human and animal. For a moment, imagine stepping into a home with draping cobwebs so dense you think they're curtains. Under your feet is literally two to three feet of animal feces and human trash. As you step in you can smell strong fumes of ammonia from urine through your mask. Taking tentative steps out of caution, you're worried that the surface below may drop out from under you or an aggressive dog with shiny white and sharp teeth will make a sudden appearance. You inch your way slowly through muck to a back bedroom in an effort to locate several pets needing an observational evaluation.

In the bedroom there are video boxes strewn in towering high piles on the dresser and a small table where a large television covered in dirt, dust, and who knows what else. The sheets are filthy with dirt on the unmade bed with two soiled pillows placed to support one's body while watching TV. You observe several dogs quivering with fear as they huddle as far back as they can in a closet with dirty, crumpled clothes spilling out. Stooping low while looking ahead, you ease out the room while holding a metal clipboard covering half your bottom in case one of the dogs decides to lunge out to bite because you'd rather get bitten than a face full of those thick cobweb curtains.

That scenario was a typical scene when called out to help people and pets caught in tough situations. What this story also represents is how our surroundings, whether that be our physical or social circles affects our physical, mental, and emotional well-being. It's not uncommon to see that many people living in clutter and filth have physical, mental, and emotional issues. When watching the television program, *Hoarder's*, you'll notice that hoarders hold onto objects because they feel abandoned or are grieving a loved one. Oftentimes, they collect animals to feel loved. Their hoarding behavior is an extreme coping mechanism for their emotional distress. For both humans and animals, an unhealthy environment affects all aspects of being a live, sentient being.

I encourage you to take a look around you. Do you have piles of papers, mail, and books on every flat surface? Are your things disorganized? Our culture encourages the purchase of a lot of needless stuff to fill our homes. Do you really need whatever you own or purchase?

Clutter is often a reflection of what's going on in our minds as an emotional coping mechanism. Messiness aside, what about cleanliness? How do you feel in your home and work areas? If you're noticing that you feel ill in any space at home or work, then consider hiring a mold specialist to inspect your home or work environments. The expense and willingness to consider your environment is worth your health.

Our experience with mold in our home invited us to do a major declutter. The process was cleansing and freeing. Room by room we made our way asking these questions about each item:

1. When was the last time I used this? More than a year — gone!
2. Is this sentimental? If yes, how do I want to preserve/display it
3. What can be donated?
4. Can this go in the dumpster? No dilly dallying on this. We went with our intuition and got it done.

The rewards of decluttering and embracing minimalistic habits are that our home is much easier to keep clean and tidy. Much time and expense went into remediating, which we'd prefer not to ever go through again. Committing to and maintaining an environmentally healthy home made perfect sense.

After significant decluttering, I went about creating relaxing and easy to tidy spaces throughout the house. Placing items that truly sparked joy where they were easily and visually enjoyed along with cozy blankets, pillows, and low lighting made each room feel inviting and warm.

As my grandmother grew older, she often gifted me with beloved treasures. Silver platters, crystal bowls, jewelry, and cooking tools. Every morning I have my coconut yogurt with blueberries from a small crystal bowl in memory of our special relationship. Memorable dishes and trinkets don't need to be squirreled away. Use them with love as they were intended to be.

We can't forget about decluttering the digital world and internet. Smartphones, apps, and the internet are designed to be addictive. Those notification pings and time-consuming scrolling are distracting, mindless, and most importantly energy depleting.

Like a majority of people, my personal and work cell phones used to be constantly pinging — texts and emails indicating a problem needed attending to at the very moment. Gone are the days of just the telephone and snail mail. The 24/7/365 requests increase with our reinforcement of a consistent immediate response. Many holidays, days off, and date nights with my husband were ruined because I was always preoccupied with something else. I believed shutting down my phones wasn't permissible. Always making myself available led to a point where I'd have visceral reactions whenever my phone pinged. I still see my husband's scowl of disappointment as our date night dinner was yet again interrupted. A night carved out for just the two of us that I ruined by being ruled by my phone. Not exactly a relationship booster, right?

In addition to decluttering and cleaning up our physical and digital spaces, we need to take a look at our social circles, too. Social circles, be they family, friends, or work-related, are also considered part of our environmental exposure that affects our overall well-being. Relationships can be supportive, neutral, toxic, or abusive. We find safety, along with support, in our social groups. As human beings we naturally want to be part of a group. The thing is that we can shape our social circles to be ones that are safe and supportive. Adjust your own social network to one that's mutually energizing and supportive. Who you include in your circle matters if you want to feel supported and safe. Distance yourself from those who drain your energy. Invite those in who show support without judgment. Quietly cull those who don't light you up off your social media platforms. There's no need to make a scene. Unfriend and block are your best friends.

Forcing yourself to belong or fit in prevents you from being your authentic self. Blending in is a form of manipulation. Being authentically you is important because to morph yourself into someone you're not is energetically draining. For a long time, I'd loyally cling to certain friends by bending over backwards to please them by buying special gifts, doing whatever they asked of me, and being generous with my knowledge, time, and money. I acted this way because I wanted to fit in, avoid rejection, and bullying. I gave all of myself only to rarely receive the same support that I handed out like candy. My behavior habit of people pleasing certainly didn't earn me long-term, valued relationships.

As I cleaned up my physical space, gained control over my digital response, and cultivated a social group that's non-judgmental, caring, energizing, and safe a sense of calm and ease filled my environment. Creating physical and social environments that are healthy and establishing boundaries around your space, time, and digital interference will relieve a lot of stress that's pushing you out of a healing state.

MINDSET

What you think truly matters. Thinking patterns and habits affect your emotions, actions, and your recovery. The mental self is your mental resilience and well-being. It's about managing your brain by making intentional choices about what you choose to believe and how you choose to treat yourself when you crash, make a mistake, or set out to achieve a dream.

Managing thoughts that your brain offers to you is possible. Learning how to manage my mind changed everything for me — my relationships, my health, my life — for the better. We all have inner voices in our heads judging, criticizing, and warning us NOT to entertain that new idea. This is normal and you don't have to let your inner voices control you anymore. Those inside voices were created by social conditioning, a comment given, or a line read in a book. Think of those beliefs as an invitation rather than a given. Invites are more easily turned down than agreeing to a belief at face value. Believing and taking hold of thoughts that aren't helpful lead to emotions that make us feel awful and ignite a maladaptive stress response that keeps the body overworking and depleting energy stores. This cycle of our thoughts and emotions affect how you evolve, how you care for yourself and others, your energy levels, and recovery.

Before making the connection between my chronic fatigue and frequent crashes, I discovered cognitive-based life coaching methods that focus on becoming aware of your thoughts and feelings. What you think about what's happening inside or outside of you is an interpretation your brain is offering to make sense of the circumstance. In turn, thoughts initiate emotions. Likewise, emotions also trigger thoughts. Together, your thoughts and feelings drive you to react or behave in a certain way. At the end of this cycle, you created a result that reflects your entire thought and all your feelings about a circumstance. For example, I was told I was healthy and that I must simply be 'one of those people' who is tired all the time. Because I was told my symptoms weren't real, I thought no one believed me, which made me feel unworthy of being heard. At the time, that thought and feeling combination built my desire to push through, overachieve, and people please to make my mark in the world.

As I did my work exploring, examining, and questioning my thoughts and beliefs I began to feel better — emotionally and physically. By shifting my perspective about myself and capabilities, I felt a calmness take over my mind and body. No more frenzied thinking or feeling wired, overwhelmed, and confused. Calmness sent my body into a healing state, offered quality sleep, refilled my energy, and gave me a calm confidence to advocate for myself that ultimately led to finding the perfect health care team.

EMOTIONAL RESILIENCE

We're socially conditioned to always be happy, tuck emotions away, and never to make a scene. Societal expectations differ whether you're female or male. Females are expected to dress appropriately by not showing too much skin, not be bold or loud, and be skinny with long legs, to name just a few. Males are also subjected to societal rules. After all, boys aren't supposed to cry, must play sports, and "man up" during difficult times. The underlying messages program us to believe it's not appropriate to feel emotions and be ashamed if we don't meet societal or familial expectations. We're programmed to believe that emotions are bad and should be hidden.

You might feel the frustration, unworthiness, and anger behind those expectations yet tamp down those emotions to show up exactly as expected. What we're not told is that it's okay to feel our emotions, let alone how to feel them. We are conditioned to have certain beliefs and expectations.

Humans feel emotions in the body, not the brain. They're nothing to be afraid of and are beneficial when embraced. The human body is exquisite in its ability to process emotions and heal the body. I understand the fear of thinking emotions will get worse rather than better, but I assure you the opposite is true. Shoving away your emotions creates a stressful environment within your body that interrupts healing and depletes your energy stores.

Everyone experiences small traumas or challenging life events. Divorce, moving from one city to another, loss of a loved one, bullying, unprovoked comments, and negative experiences are examples of challenging life events. These types of events are quickly processed, glossed over, pushed away, or tightly held onto. One day a similar event, thought, or emotion triggers discomfort that's suppressed by keeping busy, pushing through, and numbing out with food and alcohol. These tightly held emotions stack up like dinner plates until one of the plates triggers an avalanche of an emotional response that topples the entire tower down.

Tending to our small emotional wounds rather than dismissing them offers the body an opportunity to process, digest, and metabolize the metabolic waste emotions create. Emotions are sensations created by biochemical reactions within the body. Emotions are energy in motion. When you ignore and tuck away emotions, they get stuck and pile up. Back in the day when I was a massage therapist, we had a saying that we push "issues in the tissues." The kneading and deep stroking of massage helps move along the metabolic waste piling up in your muscle tissue. Emotions are signals between the body, brain, and environment communicating amongst each other. Our thinking habits, including our interpretations of an emotion, can either help or hinder emotional processing.

The willingness to have the courage to feel and process emotions offers supportive healing to your entire being — body, mind, heart, and soul. Exploring my own thinking and behavior patterns and their effect on my emotions had me not only shifting perspectives, but also feeling consistently more energetic. Addressing my mindset and emotional heart, I ignited my healing by getting quality rest, reducing stress, and building restorative energy from within.

I want you to know that you are not making up your symptoms. You are not a hypochondriac. You are not insane. You are not broken. You ARE fatigued. Tucked away emotions, along with unhelpful and unconscious thinking habits, keep the fatigue cycle going.

THE FORMULA FOR RECOVERY

The solution toward recovery is a holistic and integrative approach with a simple model that guides your healing from an objective point of view. All four factors must be addressed and ruled out. Your physical and environmental selves are priority factors. The doctors — conventional, functional, naturopathic — have your physical health side covered. Clean up your space to reduce clutter and dirt or hire someone to do it. Consider a new job or working with a relationship coach or therapist to help you make your home and work environment as healthy and supportive as possible. Maintaining a home that's clutter free keeps allergens at a minimum. Got toxic mold in your home? Hire certified professionals to remove all contaminated material, repair leaks, and rebuild or find a new non-toxic, healthy home. All these pieces and parts make a difference in your overall well-being. Get on treatment, examine your environment in place first then address those thoughts and emotions.

I invite you to consider an approach of looking at chronic fatigue from a lens that includes the above factors that impact chronic fatigue with a scientific method. When performing a scientific experiment, you first decide on a series of variables to test. The important piece is to test ONE variable at a time. For example, let's look at the variable applicable to chronic fatigue:

- PB = Physical Body: Includes viruses, infections, toxins, and genetic factors
- EE = Environmental Exposure: Includes the toxicity and stress levels within your physical and social/work environments
- M = Mindset: Includes thinking patterns that are helpful or not helpful
- ER = Emotional Resilience: Includes your awareness and willingness to work with your emotions

PB + EE + M + ER = optimal health (energy increasing)

Reflect on each variable for you. Rate each one on a scale of 0 to 10. 0 = no energy leaks to 10 = highest energy leak

Where do you need attention? Adjust one variable at a time to determine what's helping and what's not.

The main focus on illness healing is focused on ridding the body of pathogens using medications, supplements, and herbal treatments, along with physical therapy, acupuncture, massage, or energy work. This aspect is indeed very important yet there are missing variables to the formula. Two major variables for recovering from chronic fatigue is addressing and healing your 'other' inside world — your mind and emotions.

Thoughts and emotions are often taken for granted or stuffed *waaaay* down into a pit with hopes they never rise up. We all want a magic pill solution, but there isn't one. In reality, the magic pill solution is addressing your physical body, environmental exposures, mindset, and emotional resilience. Dismissing mindset and emotional wellness depletes energy, interrupts healing, encourages anxiety, and keeps the fatigue cycle rolling onward.

The truth is that you can and are meant to live a full life, even if you have an autoimmune disease you'll carry for life. Anxiety can be leveled. Calmness and clarity emanating with energy is available to you.

Three

Behind the Scenes

It's not often one gets a glimpse behind the scenes, especially when it comes to our own physical body. Once I had a basic understanding of the mechanisms contributing to the chronic fatigue cycle, it gave me space to know chronic fatigue from an objective perspective. I've always been curious about what makes living beings tick inside and out. What's happening beneath the surface, in the mind, and why people and animals do what they do. Curiosity has always led me to something new and exciting. As a massage therapist, and later a biology and neuroscience student, I learned the intricacies and complexities of the human body. My massage therapy studies especially held an unusual and exciting opportunity behind a closed door in a University of Rhode Island research department.

Stepping into the examination room, a body under a white sheet waited for us. The person laying underneath that sheet gifted her body to science for doctors to gain knowledge to better help those in need in the future. The students stood around the deceased person while holding hands and bowing their heads for a soft-spoken prayer of gratitude in honor of this gift before we were introduced to every physical detail the eye could see. Everyone was thankful and excited to dissect deeper into the body to observe and notice in awe the wonders of the human body. Observing the human body in this way gave me a deep appreciation for the impact that massage techniques have on the muscles and organs enclosed by muscle and bone.

The human body is exquisite in design. All of our organs are surrounded by fat, muscle, and bone. The nervous system connects the brain to our organs and muscles. The body and the brain work together by communicating via the nervous system highway through biochemical reactions. Lots of zings, zaps, and zips are required ingredients for us to function in terms of movement, processing nutrients and our experiences, and eliminating microscopic invaders inside the body.

Thinking about the nervous system, I envision a map showing the destinations an airline offers around the world. The lines crisscross and stop at different locations across the world according to the ticketed destination. Now, let's make that map interactive. The lines on the map light up as each flight takes off, travels toward its destination, and finally lands. The more air traffic there is the more that map lights up. Delays, interruptions, and the system starts to overheat.

All those flashes of lights indicating the path an airplane is traveling on symbolizes our nervous system collecting data from what's happening around and inside of us. The more stimulation, the more messages need to be delivered.

Those tingles, vibrations, and even aches and pains are signals that the body is doing its job. The problem is the body and brain are like two squawking blue jays yacking at full volume but not listening to each other.

Repetitive zaps of biochemically induced electrical messages zing throughout the body. Mostly these sensations and communications are automatic, unnoticed, but necessary to breathe, circulate blood, and digest our food. We rev up messages by letting mental chatter and emotions rule our day. This can feel like being wired or, on the other side of the spectrum, numb. If you're feeling wired your body is overheating itself working overtime trying to fight or flee from a perceived threat. Imagine the flight path dashboard fully and brightly lit. If you're feeling numb, then your navigation system is offline and frozen in place with no lights showing the flight path. You're shut down.

In the animal behavior world, behavioral ecology studies how animals interact with the environment, each other, and other species. Survival requires fitness — the ability to reproduce, raise, and care for the offspring, hunt or forage for food and water. An animal's instinct is to manage their energy to be sure they can outrun prey and predators by budgeting their energy to hunt for food, court mates, reproduce and care for offspring, and play to teach their offspring hunting skills. Little, if any energy, is expended for frivolousness or they won't survive. A persistent state of fear, anxiety, and anger depletes energy, interrupts a healing state, and is not ecologically economic for neither animal nor you.

The job of our nervous system is to warn us of dangers, just like our wildlife friends. The problem is that our brain hasn't evolved for our modern times. We no longer have to worry that a pride of lions plans to chase us down for a tasty meal. Without doubt, I will tell you that there are times you are in grave danger. Have you ever stepped into a room or elevator or stood next to someone who gave you the heebie jeebies? That's the same GPS system warning you of fictional danger, too. The human nervous system doesn't filter out what's real or not real, which is why everything feels real. Prey animals, such as deer, lift their heads, alert to sounds, sniff the air, and evaluate the environment to determine whether the feeling they sensed truly meant danger before fleeing. They do this because they know that persistent fear is not sustainable in the long run.

We can't forget that we're part of the great Animal Kingdom. The *Homo sapiens* brain — that's us! — evolved from our nomadic ancestors but we were gifted with a prefrontal cortex and complex linguistic areas that team up with our primitive hindbrain. That's why we have language and the ability to solve complex problems. Without the exquisite nature of the human brain, we wouldn't have landed on the moon, created life-saving vaccines, and mind-boggling computer systems. Our brain is our most valuable asset. If we use it.

The brain and body alerting to changes in our environment also applies to you and me. Neurochemicals are released when the brain and body senses an association or pattern out of the norm. Those neurochemicals are the messengers shouting the alarm, "danger, danger, danger!" when a pattern is off kilter. Our brain alerts us to changes for us to assess, filter, and determine whether action is required. The brain inadvertently allows thoughts to run rogue quickly, leading us to believe we have no control. The thing is that we do have control. The prefrontal cortex is our logic center that is a master at problem solving.

The initial intention of an alert is to prepare the body for protection and return to safety as quickly as possible then drop down to homeostasis. All attention goes to fighting or escaping so the body empties out (think Irritable Bowel Syndrome) to get you the heck out of dodge without carrying excess baggage. Your nervous system is designed for intermittent stress, which is a healthy and normal human response. But continuously being on alert is not sustainable because a maladaptive stress response that's depleting energy has been created.

Stress. We all know about stress and the importance of stress reduction. Running yourself ragged to meet the needs of everyone else except yourself, to gain more accolades, and ruminating about all that's ever gone wrong in life are weakening your nervous system and inviting infections and toxins to take up residence.

Chronic stress weakens the immune system because the associated unhelpful thoughts and feelings of fear and anxiety keep the nervous system in high alert mode. The human body is designed for occasional bursts of stress, not a constant stream. Chronic stress depletes your energy stores — physical, mental, and emotional energy — eventually making the body vulnerable to illness, pathogens, and adrenal fatigue.

Our physical, mental, and emotional well-being is vital to our level of healthy fitness. That's what this book is all about. Once you have clarity about what's happening behind the scenes, focus on cooling off your nervous system by dialing in your alert system and cultivate a care-tending routine that alleviates fatigue and your body can do the physical healing it needs.

FANNING THE FLAMES

Clearly, how we interpret what's happening inside and outside of ourselves plays a major role with the thermostat of your nervous system. Unrelenting anxiety, fear, frustration, and worry sends the nervous system into high alert mode and drives the maladaptive stress response to continually fight and protect. Negative thoughts and emotions send messages to your primitive brain center that triggers a cascade of messages alerting your body and brain to be on the lookout for danger. Sounding the alarm on a perceived threat leads you to fight, flee, or hunker down.

Threats, perceived or real, invoke thoughts and emotions in us. Without assessment, the threat messenger starts a cascade of false information. Further down at the cellular level, our unconscious, threat-evoking thoughts and dismissed emotions trigger a maladaptive stress response to be signaled by our mighty mitochondria, which are powerhouse organelles found in our cells. Mitochondria serve an additional role by acting as the signaler of cellular danger. Cell danger response researcher, Robert K. Naviaux, explains in his report, *"Perspective: Cell Danger Response Biology — The New Science That Connects Environmental Health With Mitochondria And The Rising Tide of Chronic Illness*, that the mitochondria are responsible for the physiological response to stress, which is called a cell danger response. An infection, exposure to chemicals, toxic mold, physical trauma, and our thoughts and emotional capacity trigger the cell danger response. Naviaux's research suggests that the cell danger response remains in threat mode until the mitochondria is given an "all clear" signal from affected cells. Until the "all clear" signal is received, the cell danger response continuously loops. This repetitive loop is often described as a maladaptive stress response, which interrupts and prevents healing. The cell danger response, along with its friend the maladaptive stress response, interrupts healing and leaves behind long-term chronic fatigue and diseases, such as rheumatoid arthritis, fibromyalgia, ADHD, CFS/ME, autoimmune diseases, food allergies, irritable bowel syndrome, and gluten intolerance to name a few.

Naviaux describes the cell danger response as having "...the power to change human thought and behavior, child development, physical fitness and resilience, fertility, and the susceptibility of entire populations to disease." The cell danger response can explain why sometimes you feel better but then have a crash after physical activity or an emotional upset. Stories we tell ourselves induce anxiety and stress that amplify body aches, pain, fatigue, and restlessness. We all know that the discomfort of searing hot feet means you shouldn't have walked down to the mailbox or taken the dogs for a forest walk, right? With unmanaged brain and emotional processing in place, we end up beating ourselves up for taking a short walk that keeps the cell danger response sending out a threat message.

Ruminating in the storyteller mind and the dismissed emotions fan the flames of your already overworking nervous system. Your battery is nearly depleted as you fall for the lies that you're not good enough and you don't matter. The truth is that you are good enough, you do matter, you can heal, and you can regain your energy.

The cell danger response is an important piece of research to consider in solving the chronic fatigue cycle and other illnesses. The body is designed to heal, but we need to help it out. Naviaux's work clearly suggests that how we fuel our bodies, the impact of our environment, the power of our thoughts, and the need to heal emotional wounds are all necessary to break the chronic fatigue loop triggered by the cell danger response. Taking a cue from our wild animal counterparts, reconnecting the body and brain back together, plus feeling whatever you're feeling, is part of the equation to reset, recharge, and kiss fatigue goodbye.

～ Four ～

Why You're Still Tired Yet Wired

A key clue to chronic fatigue is that you're tired yet wired in between feeling okay and in crash mode. The wired component of fatigue makes you feel restless. You can't stop moving. Restlessness while fatigued is a sign that your systems — body, mind, and emotions — are running on overdrive.

There are many ways to become chronically fatigued. Fatigue is usually first noticed after an illness where your body becomes overwhelmed by a virus, bacteria, or toxin overload. Or perhaps after a traumatic or challenging life experience. At times fatigue suddenly shows up out of nowhere. What I've come to learn and understand is that our thinking, behavior, emotional habits, and experiences all play a role in chronic fatigue. How we think, respond, and feel on a regular basis impacts the nervous system, which can increase your vulnerability to infections, inflammation, and fatigue.

There are no clear answers on whether fatigue, infection, or inflammation come first or are part of the full package. What's becoming clearer is that our body becomes vulnerable to infections and fatigue with chronic stress and challenging life events like losing a job, getting divorced, the death of a loved one, moving to a new state, or being bullied.

Fatigue is your body's way of asking for rest. We often ignore the rest signal because our world runs 24/7/365. Sleep can wait because there's more important things to get done. Pushing through fatigue became a dirty little habit of mine. And the one that plummeted me out the airplane door without a parachute. I truly get the pressure we put on ourselves and the perceived pressure we take on.

You're on proper medical treatment to eliminate or greatly reduce the load of viruses and bacteria in your body. But you're still so very tired yet wired at the same time.

What we think about creates emotions that impact how we physically feel. Likewise, emotions also create thoughts that impact how you physically feel. You're not getting better because of your thinking, or your emotional and behavior habits. Each of these areas drive energy in either a maladaptive stress response or healing response loop and play a major role in the recovery process.

There's more to the thinking thing. How you think and feel about all areas of your life affect your inner state. Is your thinking creating a lot of emotions like anxiety, worry, overwhelm, and frustration or it is driving you to push through fatigue? Thinking, as well as emotional and imbalanced behavior habits, keeps the body in a chronically stressed state that overworks and interrupts the healing process.

How you think and feel about yourself and others also plays a role in recovering. Do you tend to help others even when you really want to say no? Are you seeking perfection or driving hard to get that promotion? Do you bend over backwards to make everyone happy?

What you think about what's happening around and inside you creates emotions that drive your body to be in a healing state or a chronically stressed state and results in you either getting well or not.

The brain and body work in partnership. Relying on only external treatment protocols, such as medication, supplements, herbals, meditation, and yoga, only covers part of the solution. Inner work needs to be done to recover or find yourself in remission more often. Inner work includes resetting the nervous system and cell danger response by rewiring your brain and body by paying attention to thinking patterns, balancing your behavior habits, tending to emotional wounds, and renovating your response to situations outside and inside of yourself. Tending to these areas helps you find the calm necessary for your body to return to homeostasis and effective healing.

Five

The Influence of Your Behavior Habits

We often take small comments or advice given by others to heart. A high school guidance counselor once told me that I'd never be successful in Biology. He suggested I sign up for business classes instead. I was disappointed but did as told because I wasn't one to buck the system. The words my guidance counselor said took up residence in my head. What I really heard was that I wasn't smart enough and girls don't do science. Or maybe it was past acquaintances and role models that kept reminding me how I wasn't cut out for college. Remembering this, my Inner Rebel set out to prove them all wrong when I started college in my early 30's.

Setting out to prove to someone else wrong invites an eventual fall out. Rather than sticking to a typical semester class load, I overfilled my schedule with all but one or two classes that weren't science related. Because I entered college at a late age (at least in my mind), I pushed to complete my degree as soon as possible. This pattern repeated itself in graduate school and later in my professional life. Burning the candle at both ends, carrying a big workload, and pushing to complete projects with a final and tidy red bow were how I tackled my work. This life and work pace was a big contributor to my fatigue crashes after the challenging divorce of my first marriage, completion of my degrees, and personal and professional areas where I ignored the signals my body was sending.

My pattern of overachieving and overworking continued in my chosen career and hobby as I aged. My behavior habits of overachieving, obliging, and helping followed me wherever I went and whatever I was doing. The needle on the spectrum of my behavior habits was so off the charts that my body literally gave in.

My aim in this chapter is to share how our natural dispositions — our behavior habits — set our nervous system on fire, leave you vulnerable to disease and fatigue, and orchestrate the chronic fatigue cycle toward collapse. The behavior habits I describe reflect and add onto groundwork set by Alex Howard of the *Optimum Health Clinic* in considering personality habits that tax the chronic fatigue cycle.

Every single one of us is born with our own distinct behavioral repertoire. There is nothing inherently wrong with our behavior patterns. The problem arises when our behavior habits become imbalanced by taking them to the far end of the spectrum. We're like snowflakes shaped in differing and beautiful designs. Our behavior habits help shape our identity. They are who we are. The important bit is to understand that these pieces of us, when imbalanced, are energy depleting. Becoming aware of when and how they show up for you helps dial down your approach so you're conserving, not spending, energy.

Overall, the seven behavior habits aren't troublesome at all. We need the Chameleons because of their talent of participating on both sides to act as a diplomat. The Obligers simply want people to feel good about themselves. An innate sense of compassion is the spotlight for Helpers while the Perfectionists want to ensure their work has the greatest impact for all. We need the Achievers for innovation and growth. Even Worriers offer an opportunity to plan for potential worst-case scenarios in the event an alternative plan is needed. Last but not least, the Dramatist is an expert at gathering information that could be useful for the community.

Our behavior habits become problematic when one or more land on the spectrum of extreme. You may identify with one or many of these habits. Consider which ones you may be taking to the extreme level? Where does your desire lie to blend in, oblige, help, perfect, achieve, worry, or be involved?

CHAMELEON

Chameleons are magical reptilian creatures. They're magical because of their unique ability to change the color of their body. Unlike the gorgeous and colorful plumage of many bird species, such as peacocks and hummingbirds, whose feather colors and iridescent are worn 24/7, chameleons aren't so fortunate. In any ordinary moment, the chameleon sports a greenish outfit. She'll adjust her outfit color as the lighting, temperature, and her mood dictate. Despite popular belief, chameleons don't change color in order to blend into the environment, but that's certainly what some humans do.

Many of us do our best to blend into our social environments, whether that's our personal or work circle or both. Humans by nature want social connection, even if you're a dedicated introvert. We all want to belong to a group, to be part of social circles. But when you ignore your true self in order to fit in with a social, cultural, or work group, you do so at the cost of your well-being.

Blending and morphing ourselves to fit in with a certain crowd just doesn't feel good. Spending years of pretending to be someone else you end up feeling a loss of yourself. This is exactly what I've done in the past. Becoming who you aren't, you end up doing what you don't want to do for the sake of belonging and approval. In return you end up miserable, unhappy, alone, and without a genuine, trusting, and supportive network. The unhappiness, lack of trust, and safety in the relationship or group eventually takes a toll on your health.

You might identify with the Chameleon if you have a tendency to allow others to make decisions for you, agree when you don't agree, dress in clothes you aren't comfortable in, remain silent when you disagree, and go to great lengths to hide who you really are. Dismissing what you like, value, and experience, you are essentially dismissing yourself. And your body knows it.

We all have different talents and gifts but often we hide them from everyone else for the sake of fitting in. We often feel ashamed for doing what we're supposed to do and not what we want. Acknowledging and playing to your gifts and talents takes away angst and anxiety that align with what's right for you. There are family lineages of physicians, carpenters, shop owners, dentists, engineers, etc. This generational line up of professionals is honorable and often expected. Following in the family footsteps is terrific but only if that's what you truly want to do. Otherwise, you're fooling yourself and building up unprocessed emotions that will run you down.

We learn this skill when we're in middle school where categorization begins — the in-crowd, jocks, geeks, and nobody's. This is the time when we don't really know who we are but have ideas. To avoid bullying or being ousted, you start to morph yourself into those you surround yourself with. You might select trying to fit in with the popular girls because you want to be seen yet are dreadfully uncomfortable with the judgment that comes along with belonging to this group. You then become judgmental of others, too, because all your peers are doing the same thing.

We take this hard-earned skill to our own social circles and work environment. We bend, flex, and merge ourselves into the culture in order to be seen, heard, and get a promotion. The thing is that deep down your body knows this sleight of hand trick and doesn't like it. By not being true to yourself, the body rebels because it feels unsafe, unsupported, and unheard. A mirror reflection of the thoughts you tamp down.

Take a moment to think about how you do your best to blend in. Ask yourself these questions if you tend to flex and bend in order to fit into social circles:

- How do you change your behavior to blend in?
- What thoughts show up as you bend and flex your way into belonging?
- How does that feel in your body?

For me there is a feeling of constriction in my throat and chest and a buzzy sensation in my arms, hands, and fingers. Kind of sounds like anxiety, doesn't it? Now ask yourself these questions:

- How do you behave toward others when you're trying to belong in certain social circles?
- What do you notice — thoughts, feelings, actions — when you are truly part of a social circle?
- Which feels better? When you're a Chameleon or yourself and why?

Giving yourself permission to be you realigns and reconnects the mind and body. This is the place peace, focus, and freedom lie. Honoring and growing the gifts bestowed to you offers a sense of safety, support, and security to your entire nervous system. Anxiety and confusion fade into the background as you begin to feel at peace, focused, and at ease. Now, this isn't to say that there will never ever be a stressful moment. Your body is best equipped to handle periodic short-term stress.

Being a Chameleon has its benefits. Chameleons make good leaders and diplomats because they're able to gather information from both sides without judgment then form a consensus that will work for most everyone involved.

Chameleons, birds, and animals of all sorts don't try to blend in to be part of a group. They're either in or out. If they've been accepted into the social group, the social hierarchy is played out and each animal plays their part. If one doesn't get accepted into the group, the rejection letter is not taken personally. Instead, the ousted one heads out to find a welcoming group.

OBLIGER

You walk in the door to find that someone had a pillow fight and party while you were out shopping. Plants have been overturned and pillow fluff is all over the place. To top off the mess there is a big poop in front of the door. Mila, your playful mutt, squirms almost belly down on her way to greet you. Her tail is thumping loudly on the floor while she's yawning and trying hard to jump but yet not jump on you to plant slobbery kisses on your face as you're scolding her. Is she apologizing for her mess? Telling you she's the guilty one? Or groveling in an attempt to calm down your anger?

From a dog behavior professional point of view, Mila is doing her best to calm YOU down. Canine cognition scientists have yet to determine if dogs indeed show emotions like guilt or shame, but we can at least say she's responding to your reaction about the mess. Of course, she had a ton of fun while you were gone. Her misbehavior is reflective of boredom or, depending on the severity of damage, an indication of separation distress or anxiety.

Can you see yourself doing this? Trying to please or make someone feel happy mainly because you don't want controversy, want to be included, or liked?

Way back in the days when a 10-year-old could roam the neighborhood, the gardens and wildflowers were a prime invitation for bouquets of flowers to be picked and arranged. Every summer my mother was presented with bouquets of handpicked flowers. To this day I still buy her flowers or create handpicked bouquets from my own garden. Yes, I want to please my mother but my intention in my fresh handpicked flower bouquets were always about sharing my love.

On the other end of the spectrum, what about gift giving to a mentor or friend as a token of their acceptance? What if you spent quite a bit of money on a gift only for that person to say a quick thanks and set that gift aside? And then later discover they gave that gift to someone else?

Offering to take on tasks or our generosity when we're tired, want a break, time for ourselves, or just don't want to do it — we do those things to please the person without considering our own needs.

Saying yes all the time makes it hard to say no when you really need or want to. People expect you to say yes when yes is always your response. You could be flat on your back with exhaustion and flu-like symptoms, yet you get up, get dressed, and head out the door when they come calling.

What if I told you that being an Obliger is manipulation? Pure and simple manipulation. You're trying to manipulate a person to like you by bending over backwards without any boundaries to support you. When you say yes to someone else, you're telling you and your needs a big fat no. Are you inwardly saying no when you say yes? How are you saying no to you when you say yes to someone else? What is the benefit to you if you said no?

Once I learned that Obligers are manipulators, I began to pay close attention about why I wanted to say yes to a person or activity. I get it, saying no is hard at first but with practice becomes easier. The first time I finally said no it felt like a 200-ton weight lifted off my back. Each subsequent no became easier. Now, I take a pause to think about whether I truly want to say yes or no before making any commitment.

Are you always giving rather than receiving? Explore being an Obliger with the following questions:

- Why do I feel the need to give and please others?
- What am I afraid of if I don't?
- How do I feel inside when I give more than I receive?
- What am I saying yes to that I really want to say no to?

Being an Obliger is a huge energy expense with little to nothing in return. You can't keep giving if your energy cup is low or virtually empty. When you start saying no to those things you don't want to do, energy generates so that what you want to do is more doable.

HELPER

In the news we hear about burnout in careers and caregiving. Many people are exhausted from their jobs or caregiving to loved ones. Burnout can cause you to fall ill, walk away from a job you enjoyed, or cause chronic fatigue bad enough that you can't care for others, let alone yourself because the energy stores are depleted. Giving more of ourselves than receiving eventually takes a physical and emotional toll that keeps the chronic fatigue cycle running.

In the animal welfare industry, workers spend years caring for animals that are homeless or victims of cruelty and neglect. Often animals of cruelty and neglect are kept in temporary housing without the option to be adopted. These cats, dogs, and horses are considered property and end up being held as live evidence, which can last several years. Caregivers may become emotionally attached to the animals they care for that they'll work for days on end without taking a day or two off to refresh and revive.

High spectrum Helpers and caregivers, no matter the industry, witness and hear trauma all the time. Emotional meltdowns, injuries, mental and physical suffering, and working long days without breaks are challenging life moments that induce emotions that need to be processed for the body to eliminate them.

These superhero, hardworking, and highly caring caregivers run the risk of succumbing to chronic or compassion fatigue. Helper fatigue comes when you give more to others than yourself until you no longer have the capacity to help. That's when you fall and fall hard. The human body cannot sustain persistent stress and challenging life moments even though our culture tries damn hard to make us believe we can.

Being a Helper is a mighty fine gift to have. The world needs people to help care for the sick, injured, and homeless. Helpers freely give their hearts to those in need. Helpers are healers, health care professionals, therapists, teachers, veterinarians, and animal welfare workers, to name a few. We need helpers to remind us about compassion.

We need helpers and fixers in the world but it's not fair nor right that you sell your soul and health to help those who need you. The energy cost to a high spectrum Helper is that you're putting the welfare and care of others well ahead of yours. Overhelping runs energy at a deficit. You're not the only one that can fix a problem. The more mentally and emotionally resilient helpers that are out there, the greater impact they have with those they care for because you have energy to spare.

If helping is one of your gifts, ask yourself:

- Why is it important for you to help the way you currently do?
- What is the cost of helping at your current level?
- What do you want your helper ways to look and feel like?
- In what ways can your helper tendencies have a greater impact by taking care of your emotional, mental, and physical needs first?

PERFECTIONIST

Perfection. There are many people who strive for perfection. Society, family, friends, bosses, co-workers, you name it, so many people expect perfection out of everyone. And, probably from themselves, too.

What is perfection? My favorite definition came from Google's Dictionary: "the condition, state, or quality of being free or as free as possible from all flaws or defects."

There is nothing in this world that is perfect. There will never be the perfect project completed, book written, job done, marriage, career, hair style, fashion, car, home, or pet. Do you even know when perfect is perfect? How do we even know where the flaws are if we keep working and working on perfecting the task at hand?

Perfection makes me think about Buzz Lightyear's proclamation, *"To infinity and beyond!"* in the movie *Toy Story*. I also fondly think about my husband entertaining our young nephew with his deep laughter while the two were watching *Toy Story* and shouting, "To infinity and beyond" together. I swear that laughing together was much more fun for all than the storyline!

"To infinity and beyond" tells me to keep on going. There's no end in sight with infinity. There's no ending or destination in sight.

Striving for infinity, or I mean perfection, means putting in all-nighters to finish a project, editing manuscripts over and over until you're forced to submit, or never finishing what you started. Perfection is stagnation.

Chasing after perfection thrives on self-criticism, questions your self-worth, and breeds anxiety and self-doubt that create indecision, overworking, and task paralysis.

Perfection also has a benefit. The drive toward perfection tends to make a person more thoughtful about how they carry out a plan. They create plans rather than shoot from the hip, and being detail oriented helps spot possible problems or entices an idea to come forward.

No matter what, when you aim for high spectrum perfection either the task remains incomplete or you're exhausted from the hours invested and worrying about imperfection or both! On top of that, you're grumpy and snarking at everyone around you while berating yourself. Persistent living in this zone is bound to wear you down and out quickly.

Absolute perfection doesn't exist. Even in nature, perfection doesn't exist.

Explore your perfectionism more closely if this is how you identify:

- What does perfection mean to you?
- What thoughts and emotions show up when you're striving for perfection?
- What is the benefit of those thoughts and emotions?
- What is the cost or what are you missing out on when you strive for perfection?

Let's look at the opposite side of the coin:

- What if you aimed for good enough?
- What if your flaws and quirks were good enough and exactly what they should be?
- How would you then feel as you now strive to complete that project?

ACHIEVER

Achievers are never satisfied with what they already know. Imposter Syndrome often drives their mission to achieve in hopes that the accomplishment proves their value and knowledge. Achievement drives you to expand your knowledge and do more in order to help and achieve more at a higher level. That drive for achievement often triggers chronic fatigue symptoms.

Overachievement masks underlying emotions that are uncomfortable along with a set of beliefs that you need to know you've succeeded. Owning a home with a picket fenced yard with 2.5 children and a dog by the time you're 30 is not a definition of success, unless you decide it is. Earning more degrees or throwing yourself into your career to climb the promotion ladder at a whirlwind pace while stepping on the toes of others because wanting to earn top dollar means success is often the match and the fuse igniting the chronic fatigue cycle.

Achievers are near and dear to my heart because I am one. My childhood was filled with everything horses, including small local horse shows. My love of horses hitched a ride when I moved away as a young married adult, where I always found a way to ride and be involved with horses. Attending a Dressage at Devon show with my mother and grandmother one year, a local group put on a demonstration of dog agility, which resembles horse show jumping events. At the time I was horse poor but had a young mixed breed dog. My first ever dog, Zippy, and I became addicted to this fun sport of dog agility together. One day I realized dog agility was a way to escape the unhealthy marriage I was in. Thus, the first chapter of my achievement addiction began.

I trained with the best trainers and coaches because I wanted to learn, grow, and win. My love for working with dogs sparked an interest in massage therapy for performance sport horses and dogs because I wanted to help keep these animals in tip top shape. Then I grew my business to include the human end of the leash and bridle. I loved my work. Discovering I had the aptitude to learn hard things, I did. A double science undergraduate major and master's degree soon followed with an intention for veterinary school, but I fell in love with the world of behavior and the mechanisms that explain why animals and humans do what we do. The stress that rides alongside the drive to achieve a double major and master's degree ignited my chronic fatigue cycle and became a habit.

Looking back, the road to achievement was a typical path. Where the path started to be overgrown with obstacles was when courses, certifications, jobs, and competitions were selected because I had to prove my knowledge and skill rather than using my education along with my heart. You don't have to allow someone else's opinion to direct what you want to achieve and do. I found a sense of calm once I chose to use my heart and not only my degrees, certifications, and competition awards. I found an uptick in creativity once I decided I wouldn't let what others "think" I should do rule my life. What I've studied, researched, and accomplished was the perfect path and applies to all that I do to this very day.

The wonderful thing about being an Achiever is that you want to grow and develop yourself. Achievers are looking for how they can better themselves. There is nothing inherently wrong with building your achievement portfolio. The way you go about building that portfolio matters to your nervous system. If you're pushing and never feeling satisfied with where you are then anxiety and urgency are building in your body like a bomb ready to blow.

Maybe you're someone like me who has achieved a lot and strives for more. If those achievements feel good deep in your soul, then you're on the right track. Exploration is warranted if you feel ashamed, like a fraud, or don't yet know enough. Someone can look you straight in the eye and tell you that you don't need that job, have too many letters after your name, the words you use are too big and it DOES NOT matter. Those comments are reflections of what they wish for themselves. You have a choice to believe that what that person says is right for you or to not believe them at all.

Achievers end up overworking and overthinking much of the time, which depletes their body of valuable energy, and often triggers a fatigue crash. Achievement can be accomplished in ways that manage your brain and body energy versus overstimulation of your nervous system, which will lead to a physical breakdown.

Questions to ask yourself are:

- Why are my achievements important to me? And, to others?
- What value do I place on achievements for myself?
- What do I benefit from with all my achievements?
- What has been/is the cost to me with my focus on achievements?

WORRIER

You can't sleep because you're running a conversation you had earlier over and over and over in your head. The scene changes as you reenact every word, sentence, and intonation. You worry about what you said, they said, and what went unsaid. Anxiety runs high as you replay that scene over and over again. You can feel the guilt, fear, or shame underneath the anxiety.

Waking up at 2 a.m. then counting the number of hours of sleep left until you have to get up for work prevents you from actually falling asleep again. Counting the hours left to sleep was a major pattern for me that prevented quality sleep. Worrying about sleep easily creates withdrawal and avoidance by declining invitations for social activities and being focused on the clock rather than a conversation with a loved one or the movie you're watching.

Fantasizing worst-case scenarios does the same thing. We worry about what our spouse and family think about a change you want to make, what bosses think of our job performance, or a miscommunication with friends. Excessive worrying turns on anxiety and fretting that trigger the chronic fatigue cycle to keep on churning. The probability is high that your worst-case scenario will never come to fruition, except only in your mind. Is it worth creating an amazing action film in your head for the angst you're putting yourself through?

Worrying about what other people will say stops you from being you, putting your work out in the world, and keeps your nervous system simmering. Of course, what some people advise may matter but you get to call the final shots. Making someone else's opinion matter much more than yours is exactly how we give our power away. You don't have to hand over your power to these fictional tales you tell yourself.

Worry can be a useful emotion that invites research into a solution rather than looking at how bad the problem seems to be. Worry becomes a problem when you allow yourself to swirl and whirl in it with overthinking and fantasizing.

Take a few moments to look at worrying more closely:

- What are you worried or anxious about?
- Why are you worried/anxious? Be specific.
- What's the worst that can happen? What emotion comes up for you?
- What's the best that can happen? How would that feel for you?
- What can you do to move toward a solution and the best that can happen?

DRAMATIST

The Dramatist is an interesting character because there are a couple of facets to being one. On one hand, a Dramatist takes on the "woe is me" outlook that leans on victimhood. On the other hand, a Dramatist is one who is an information gatherer but who is also capable of creating distrust around them. Either way, a big deal is made that depletes energy while creating a sense of distrust from within and with all the people involved.

Who doesn't love to learn about what's happening around us or hear a little bit of dirt or gossip about someone or something? It's interesting to follow the stories about celebrities, within family, our social circles, and even our neighbors down the street. Gossip is a way to communicate, especially if it's sharing goodness rather than dishing dirt. The Dramatist loves to compare themselves and others by who they think is better than themselves.

In the old days, communication about the goings on in the world, our communities, and between families was conducted by word of mouth or handwritten letters until the telephone and television were invented. Nowadays, we're fully immersed in information on a 24/7 basis through the internet and smartphones. Headlines, marketing, and communications between our social networks are often sensationalized and scrutinize any and every aspect of a person as if they're simply an object to be criticized.

Being a Dramatist means you're focused on other people's business while offering judgments about what they should be doing instead. You know what's happened and what they're doing. You are firmly in the social loop, acting like a lurking stalker behind the keyboard or around the corner. You might laugh and make jokes about their work, how they dress, what they say or don't say. Dramatists know it all and are happy to spread the news.

The problem with being a Dramatist is that you're taking on a lot of anxiety and stress. You're blowing out of proportion what someone else is doing or how they're living instead of focusing on what's best for yourself. Why is caring about how another person is living and dressing, or what they're saying or doing so important to you? What are you trying to cover up about yourself? Dramatists usually feel they're lacking in their life or they're a target for all the wrong in the world. They compare then despair what they don't have by telling themselves stories about how wrong their target happens to be by tearing them down to anyone who will listen. They often have a pity party for one inside their heads. Comparison, my friend, is a one-way ticket down the shame spiral.

Comparison is one of the top problems I help clients balance out from their Dramatist ways. One client frequently compared herself to other participants who were more successful than her. It's a "have or have not" type of mindset that's triggered by shame. She'd stand ringside giving a constant negative commentary filled with sarcastic barbs about the unsuspecting victim's integrity. Her commentary at times seemed humorous but they were invisible poisoned arrows meant to inflict harm on someone she considered better than her. She believed everyone was better than her because her autoimmune condition held her back. Her belief that she wasn't good enough because she has a health issue created a lot of shame. One of the ways she chose to numb her shame was by getting into everyone else's business, especially when they reflected what she wanted for herself. Once we spotlighted the role shame played in fueling her chronic fatigue cycle, she dumped despair and began using comparison of those she admires for inspiration. More importantly, she learned that feeling shame is okay because it will always be there.

Those invisible poisoned arrows that my client used to throw at admired colleagues are sarcasm. I've used sarcasm and I bet you have, too, at various points in your life. We often think our sarcastic remarks are humorous, but below their surface they're not funny at all. Sarcasm is an invisible shield we hold tight around ourselves to protect our vulnerabilities. Our brain thinks sarcasm keeps us safe, yet our hearts do not. The etymology behind sarcasm means to "tear flesh." Words certainly can have barbs and you never know how someone else will take those words.

One of my long-ago mentors taught all her managers to never joke or be sarcastic because you never know how those words will land on another. The receiver may even laugh along with you, you who may be oblivious to what emotions those words actually triggered for them. I recall being part of a group that tossed sarcasm around like popcorn popping uncontained over flames. Like many others, I joined in on the fun and games until one day the barbs were unexpectedly flung my way. I smiled and laughed along while pretending that their words didn't bother me at all. The old adage, "Sticks and stones may break my bones, but words will never hurt me" is a big, fat lie for many. Many people believe those stinging words. Those sarcastic barbs take hold until you truly know that your own thoughts are more powerful than the words of other people. When you fully believe thoughts are optional then those barbed words don't penetrate and, perhaps, rearrange a social circle without fuss.

Your vulnerabilities may be your shame, insecurities, your enoughness, or whether or not you matter. Those shields are held up to stop the darts shooting our way while we shoot those who reflect what we wish about ourselves. It's a war of words meant to harm. Rather than being in conflict with others, change perspectives by observing how you're inspired by that person instead.

Being a Dramatist isn't all bad news. Dramatists are savvy about gathering useful information. Think about journalists who get the inside scoop on what's happening in our world. They know who to talk to, how to sort and filter the gathered information, and then communicate what they've learned for the benefit of others. Dramatists are the communicators in the world.

Plain and simple, your business is your business. Their business is their business. What other people say and do is okay (unless they're about to seriously harm someone!). Minding your own business dials down the drama dramatically while halting the chronic fatigue cycle. Save your vulnerabilities for friends who are worthy of your stories. Not everyone needs to or should have access to your most personal thoughts and feelings. Nor should you be privy to somebody else's.

It's bad enough that our out-of-balance behavior habits rev up our nervous system. Getting involved in someone else's business ramps it up even more.

Ask a few questions when you find yourself getting into somebody else's business:

- Do I need to know this? Why or why not?
- Why is it important for me to share this information with others?
- What's my intention behind sharing this information?
- What am I making the action or words of another mean about me?

In general, these behavior habits are parts of who we are. They're often our strengths and dictate why we choose the careers and hobbies that we do. Intrinsically, they aren't bad in and of themselves. The extreme versions do have an effect on our health by keeping the nervous system stimulated, overworked, and provide the chronic fatigue cycle momentum.

These behavior habits are representative of the ways that we hide, stay small, and contain emotions. Each one has a distinct path, hoping that it will lead to emotional safety but it never does. Designing a new approach to how you find your people, say yes to you first, help in a healthy, sustainable manner, accept perfect imperfections, achieve goals, find solutions, and stay in your lane soothes and heals your nervous system and chronic fatigue.

Take note of which behavior habits you're out of balance by using The Behavior Habit Energy Gauge below. Then strive to find balance!

THE BEHAVIOR HABIT ENERGY GAUGE

How much energy are you using by engaging in the Behavior Habits? Think about and imagine a specific situation where one of the behavior habits is evident. How much energy was expended? Circle how much energy is left in your tank after one or more of these behavior habits. Any behavior habit below the ½ mark is in need of balancing to reduce energy consumption.

Behavior Habit	You identify if ...	Benefit	Cost	Your Energy Gauge
Chameleon	You bend and flex yourself to fit or blend into your social circles; you make decisions based on the choices of others.	You make a great leader and diplomat. You tend to gather information before forming judgment.	You're not being true to yourself.	E ¼ ½ ¾ F
Obliger	You drop everything to complete tasks, take on more than reasonable, give gifts when not necessary, and always available to please others. Rarely, if ever, say no.	You give from the heart by thoughtfully showing love and care. You make others feel seen.	You manipulate others by demanding to be seen and heard by giving in order to belong.	E ¼ ½ ¾ F
Helper	You do anything to help out, even when you're tired or have other plans.	You show others they matter through caregiving, teaching, healing, etc.	You put others ahead of yourself.	E ¼ ½ ¾ F
Perfectionist	You work through a problem or project being as thorough as possible.	You offer well-thought out projects and plans, and are meticulous, and detail-oriented.	You question your self-worth, breed anxiety, are overwhelmed by self-doubt and anxiety.	E ¼ ½ ¾ F
Worrier	You are persistently fantasizing about worst-case scenarios.	You tend to research solutions rather than focus on the problem or negatives.	You easily send your body into a non-healing state. You hide and stay small.	E ¼ ½ ¾ F
Dramatist	You're focused on other people's business while making assumptions and gossiping.	You gather information, sort and filter what they've learned, and then communicate beneficial information.	You get caught up in the business of others in a way that causes emotional damage to everyone involved.	E ¼ ½ ¾ F

Figure 2: The Behavior Habit Energy Gauge

Six

The Effect of Your Thinking Habits

I sensed dark, stormy thunderheads hovering over me when my chronic fatigue symptoms started rising again. Wandering from ring to ring in a large indoor soccer facility watching bits and pieces of competitors running their agility I felt as though I were in a tunnel. The sounds and sights around me were muffled while only three feet ahead of me was visible. Thoughts were racing and whirling by so fast that I couldn't catch them all. Suddenly, one or two thoughts caught my attention. I grabbed and held tight onto a few thoughts my Inner Critic spoke the loudest. "I'm just not good enough" or "I'm always wrong" or "I'm invisible." Sadness, shame, and inadequacy were felt deep in my bones and soul so much so that I felt as though I was trudging through thick sludge. I got sucked into the vortex of misery, anxiety, and exhaustion by believing the stories I told myself about all the ways I've failed, wasn't good enough, and had no purpose. I felt directionless and stuck in a deep rabbit hole with no way out.

This is a perfect example of what happens when you let your brain run wild.

One of the biggest lessons I've taken away from my healing journey is that we are not our thoughts. Becoming aware and learning how to shift and manage my thinking relieved much of my underlying anxiety.

I used to push away my fatigue. For as long as I can remember my fatigue was categorized as a teenager thing, a figment of my imagination, and I was one of "those" people from the conventional medical community. Those sentiments were taken to heart. The quiet rebel in me rebelled against all those sentiments and I pushed myself until I could push no more.

Let me be clear here. There is nothing wrong with rebelling against what other people say. Implementation is what matters. See, while my body was telling me it needed rest, I pushed through to prove my worth to someone other than me. My thinking that I had to prove to a select group of people that I had the ambition and drive despite my fatigue was for them and not me. What I know now is that I can have ambition and drive in a way that supports my chronic fatigue.

Looking back, I'd trust my heart more to be me, to listen to my body instead of the words and beliefs instilled in me by external noise and the generations of women behind me.

We all have an inner GPS that leads us to what we're destined to do. This GPS system is programmed specifically for each individual person. There's a generational influence but, in general, our GPS system is specific to you. It's the part of us that lights up whenever we discover something interesting. It's why I love specific aspects of animals, art, and experiencing life and why you might not resonate with them. Too often our thinking reroutes our inner GPS, especially when influenced by outside sources.

Alongside our inner GPS, we also have a part of us that's judgmental and punitive and that's affectionately called our Inner Critic. We tend to listen to our Inner Critic, who stops us from following our heart, growing, and experiencing what we truly desire.

Our Inner Critic is that inside voice that tells you things like you're the only one with chronic fatigue, you can't make the changes you want, you'll never get better, do it right or not at all, you're not good enough, we don't talk about that, or why did you say that? These are sentences we tell ourselves over and over. Our Inner Critic is our internal judge that doesn't hold back on their judgment. Essentially, the Inner Critic causes us to punish and beat ourselves up while giving up our power to something that exists only in our minds. What's even more interesting is that we project our Inner Critic onto others, which provides us with further evidence of our self-judgment. The Inner Critic sets us up to receive exactly what we want to avoid in the first place.

The Inner Critic takes away the power we rightfully own. Our Inner Critic spoils the fun, possibilities, keeps us stuck, and dulls our shine. Engaging with our Inner Critic jumpstarts and fuels the chronic fatigue cycle.

Mindset has everything to do with your chronic fatigue recovery, including those thinking patterns running in the background undetected. These are thoughts that we've been running on for so long that they've become a habit. A habit that runs on automatic. We just do it without thinking. You don't need to think about brushing your teeth, right? You pick up your toothbrush, apply toothpaste, brush then rinse without much thought. Have you ever wondered how you got home from work some days? You don't remember the 6 stoplights or exiting off the highway. All you remember perhaps is pulling up in your driveway saying to yourself, "Well, how did I get here?" Yup. You drove home on automatic, probably lost in thought or daydreaming. The route is routine and you don't have to actively think about it.

YOU ARE NOT YOUR THOUGHTS

The thing is you are not your thoughts. Period. Thoughts are what the brain does in an attempt to associate, find patterns, and make sense of what's happening inside and outside of us. There are days I think animals are fortunate to not have such complex brains! The problem lies in that we have a tendency to attach thoughts to a story line that's not necessarily true. And yet we hold on for dear life while finding evidence to give truth to the story we've imagined.

Whatever you're thinking about you create. My horseback riding instructor used to tell me, "Wherever you're looking, your horse will go." The same adage applies here. *What you think, you create.* Let's go even deeper — *what fires together, wires together.* If you're always thinking you're not worthy, deserve to be ill, are a failure, not enough, then your brain builds neural pathways that get stronger and stronger. Pretty soon, the thought runs silently in the background, like brushing your teeth without thinking about it. That neural pathway has become a superhighway. What you're choosing to think and act upon is constructing a highway that leads far away from your desired destination.

Don't let that piece frighten you! Luckily, we have the ability to reshape our brain. Thoughts are optional and your brain can be reprogrammed by inputting intentional and helpful thoughts. You can choose what you want to believe, too. Just because society or your family chose certain beliefs, you can modify, change, or delete any belief.

Choosing your thoughts and beliefs are empowering, especially when they get you out of a rut and feeling better. We give our power away when we choose to hold onto the thoughts and beliefs that don't work for us individually. You have the power to choose thoughts that create feelings that help you get unstuck and headed in the direction you want. What beliefs do you want? Ones that limit your living and healing or ones that create growth, expansion, and recovery? The choice is truly yours.

The real truth of the matter is that you are perfect as you are, quirks and all. I believe we are here to be the best possible version of ourselves by growing, testing, and doing good in the world. We are not here to suffer. I simply don't understand why that would be the objective. Have you noticed that the great variety of animal species on this great and beautiful planet Earth don't have nearly the magnitude of problems humans do? The majority of problems animals do have are a manmade construct. How can it be that animals aren't here to suffer yet humans are?

Take a pause to grab a piece of paper or journal and a pen to do a little exploration about your beliefs:

- What do you believe? Write down all your beliefs.
- Why do you believe each one?
- List how each belief is helping you?
- List how each belief isn't helpful?
- Which ones do you want to keep? Why?

MANAGING A WILD & ROGUE MIND

Humans, like any other species, are motivated by three factors. We naturally seek pleasure, avoid discomfort, and conserve energy. This natural desire is called the Motivational Triad (Figure 2). We become experts at seeking pleasure by numbing or zoning out instead of taking control of rogue thinking. Acknowledging then focusing on intentional thinking helps calm the nervous system that interrupts the chronic fatigue cycle.

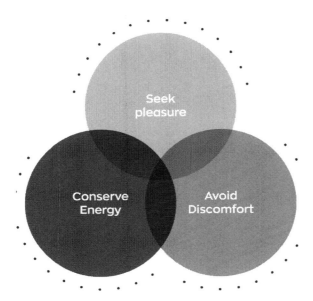

Figure 3: Motivational Triad

By the time I was diagnosed with mold illness, I was adept at creating intentional thinking. As an experiment, I decided to simply observe my unruly mind without attaching myself to any thought while in the middle of a Herximer reaction, which means the immune system is fighting off infection that makes symptoms feel temporarily worse. Laying on the sofa half-awake with *The Great British Bake Off* playing on the television in the background, my body was achy, feverish, fatigued, heavy, and anxious. Thoughts were swirling in my head and they were not happy ones, for sure. Out of curiosity, I let the thoughts run wild and unmanaged for quite some time. The longer I let those thoughts fester in my head, the worse I felt emotionally and physically. My emotions ran from anxiety, worry, and fear. My Inner Critic unleashed her punitive judgment while negative thoughts spun in my head. I got myself out of my thought spiral by recentering myself with meditation, journaling, and a nap. My experiment reminded me of the time before I started my healing journey, before I started truly exploring my thoughts and emotions.

Simply put, our thoughts create our emotions, which fuel our behavior, which triggers the chronic fatigue cycle. Likewise, what we feel creates thoughts that fuel our reaction that drive our chronic fatigue cycle. Becoming aware and intentional with our thinking habits contribute to breaking the chronic fatigue cycle.

What's not helpful is that our brain naturally pulls toward the negative. Don't be surprised when all your thinking isn't positive or pushes back when feeding it positive thoughts. Our brain has a negative bias because it's trying to protect you. When you're trying to protect a part of you, you're more prone to determining that everyone and everything is out to get you. Your brain falls for that every time with a new circumstance occurring externally or internally, a thought you're having, an emotion your body feels, or an action you take. The brain hasn't yet evolved to deal with modern day events, which are non-life threatening. Our brain is still trying to protect us from the lions, tigers, and bears — oh, my!

I want to note that there are times that our brain and body signal to us that we're in danger. Think about a time when a stranger followed too closely behind you or stepped into the elevator. The hair on the back of your neck raises, breathing slows down, and senses seem heighted. Your intuition or gut instinct were right on track and doing their job. There is a difference between your mind and body warning you of true danger and offering misinformation because it doesn't realize that asking for a promotion isn't going to kill you.

Fortunately, a few years prior to my chronic fatigue, Lyme, and mold diagnoses, I learned the power of thought work. Since I'm as curious as a marmoset and my experience debunking my thinking, I laid on the sofa taking notes. Mold has a mysterious way about it, especially the toxic water damage types of molds. Mold was invading every cell in my body, not just my sinuses and lungs. Mold was part of the reason why I frequently fell ill for over two years. Mold was taking down my immune system so, of course, I began having a lot of interesting and many unhelpful thoughts.

You don't need to have an overload of mold or virus or bacteria in your body to experience overthinking and swirling thoughts. Many women experience the same wild kind of thinking during certain periods of their menstrual cycles. However, these body invaders and fluctuating hormones have a way of amplifying negative thought loops. Ongoing thought loops, however generated, lead to mental fatigue, and mental fatigue leads to crashes.

I am grateful for the power of thought work and my love for researching or I'd probably still be sick or letting my brain rule my world. I'd be sick and miserable, which is not what I wanted in my life. Thought work or mind management has been around for ages, even since the ancient times, so this approach isn't a new, modern invention. It's a way of becoming intentional with our minds and life that we aren't taught by our families, school, or church.

Thought work is about acknowledging then letting go of unhelpful thinking. In some ways our brain isn't as smart as we think. The brain is busy looking for patterns and associations yet doesn't understand context. That's where journaling and thought work come in handy. Write out your thoughts, review what you've written, analyze the outcome of what you're thinking, then choose whether to keep or change the thought habit that has a greater cost than benefit to it. Thought work is an invitation to notice our thoughts, acknowledge both the helpful and unhelpful thoughts, filter out the unhelpful thoughts, and then detach or release thoughts that drive the chronic fatigue cycle. That's the beauty of being human. We can, indeed, become selective in our thinking habits.

Thought work can be challenging and uncomfortable, but I can assure you that nothing bad will happen to you other than an emotion. We keep ourselves distracted with shopping, eating, social media, alcohol, and a busy schedule that prevents us from slowing down because that's when the thoughts come around. I invite you to become friends with your thinking. Put on your curiosity hat and rummage around to see what is there. I promise you that curiously investigating your inner mind will shine a light on what's stopping you from healing, going for that job, career or life you've only dreamed of. Your thinking is the only thing holding you back. If you can see what's happening, then you don't have to continue doing and being what you see.

Let's shine a light on those shadowy thoughts because change is in the air and if you see those thoughts then you can heal and be fully you.

Create a daily journaling habit to write down all your thoughts. Your brain is meant to troubleshoot and process rather than act as a file cabinet. Empty out to save precious mental energy.

- Buy a journal or notebook you absolutely love
- Start with 2- or 5-minute sessions
- Ask an open-ended question, write everything your brain offers up. Everything.
    Question Examples:
    – What do I think about [circumstance]
    – How do I feel about [circumstance] or when I think [thought]
    – How do I feel about feeling [emotion]
    – What do I think about having chronic fatigue?
- Don't worry about grammar, complete sentences, or making sense
- Give yourself permission to be brutally honest

CREATING A HEALING MINDSET

Often when we start out doing something new, Imposter Syndrome, the Achiever habit, and comparison with the more experienced start controlling your thinking, emotions, and actions. My Achiever behavior habit was in full force a few decades ago when I started out as an inexperienced dog trainer and applied animal behaviorist. I was intensely aware of the successful colleagues around me. Feeling that I didn't yet know enough, I attended more courses and programs to gain more certifications to "prove" I knew my stuff. I thought, at the time, that those certifications and education would bring the people to me. I struggled growing my business while watching others create similar but more successful training and behavior consulting practices. Instead of offering my expertise to those who needed help with their pets, I chose instead to make the lack of my business growth mean that I wasn't smart enough, savvy enough, or talented enough. I felt inadequate because I wasn't as successful. Inadequacy kept me from sharing my knowledge and experience to those who needed it. I hid behind the shame of Imposter Syndrome by taking more courses, busying myself with unrelated tasks, and snacking while shopping for more courses or stuff I didn't need. My thoughts and feelings blocked me from showing up in life and business.

The truth is that I knew enough. I got swept up by my Achiever habit, comparing myself to others and cuing my brain to play stories sadly reminiscent of those childhood years of being bullied. Highlighted were all my fears, anxieties, and rejections. Distracting myself by taking more courses and spinning in confusion kept my chronic fatigue cycle running. The thing is my story is common among my clients who are out of balance with their Achiever habits.

Many of my clients think they'll always be tired and that there's no way to overcome their fatigue when they're officially diagnosed with chronic fatigue. My client, Jenny, thought there was absolutely no way she'd feel energy again when she came to me. Thinking about her chronic fatigue made her feel anxious and overwhelmed about both her personal and professional life, worried what people thought about her, whether she'd get well, and depressed that her life had become limited. Those emotions kept her on the sofa watching television when she managed to get herself up out of bed. She'd often ruminate in self-pity, which prolonged her chronic fatigue. She finally had an "aha" moment when she read an article that eventually led her to me. That article sparked enough energy for her to begin researching potential solutions. She wasn't quite ready to give up. Through our work together she redesigned her thinking and behavior habits, tended to her emotional heart, and created a new lifestyle that supported healing for her illness. Her willingness to explore her inner world turned off the cascade of events that kept her chronic fatigue cycle running on high.

Chronic fatigue isn't just about having a virus or autoimmune disease and getting medical treatment. Medical treatment is part of the equation to recovering from chronic fatigue. The chronic fatigue recovery equation is a holistic one. One that includes medical treatment, nutrition, environment, AND mindset and emotions. Allowing your mind to run wild and free while ignoring your emotions is part of the problem. Managing your mind and tending to your emotions is a big part of the solution.

An added bonus to having a high accumulation of virus, bacteria, mold, or fluctuating hormones is the occasional thought frenzy. I call them thought frenzies because suddenly the brain frantically produces thoughts. The Inner Critic is having a meltdown and tantrum. This is <insert sarcasm> delightful. I invite you to give yourself permission and space to let the thoughts fly without paying much mind to them. You do not need to listen nor attend to them. Allow this time for yourself to dive into inspirational movies, enjoy a hot Epsom bath with lavender oil, candlelight and soft music, journal, create any form of art, or read a favorite book that makes you smile.

Becoming aware, examining, and selecting helpful thoughts jumpstart your healing journey. You are not at the mercy of your brain. The choice of how you think is yours and starts with awareness of what the brain is saying. The mind and what you think affects, contributes, and sets the nervous system into a healing or non-healing state. Which will be your choice?

THE THINKING HABIT CASCADE

How do you do this, you ask? The Thinking Habit Cascade is a blueprint of a series of cascades to consider that's based on ancient beliefs about thinking, Cognitive Behavioral Therapy (CBT), Byron Katie's *"The Work,"* and *"The Model"* framework developed by a coach mentor Brooke Castillo of *The Life Coach School.* Stepping back to observe my own thinking, like the way that I've observed and evaluated animal behavior in a variety of environments from a neutral point of view, has shifted the lives of my clients and myself in creating new thinking habits that serve our lives better. The following basic Thinking Habit Cascade is flexible and helps you to objectively examine your mindset:

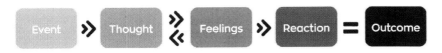

Events trigger thoughts, which in turn create feelings that drive your behavior/reaction that give you an outcome. The outcome is used as future evidence to the brain that your thought is true.

Events are circumstances and scenarios happening internally and externally to you. Events, such as a diagnosis of CFS/ME, an autoimmune disease, or something a person did or said, how you've reacted toward yourself or someone else, or even an emotion you are feeling at the very moment, trigger a thought. Consider it like a noun — a person, place, or thing. It's factual. It is what it is. Events happening inside and outside of you trigger thoughts and feelings that drive you to react. The outcome of your reaction may or may not be of service to you.

The Thinking Habit Cascade also sparks when you're having a thought that's come out of seemingly nowhere. You capture the thought first, which creates an event and then a feeling, which drives your behavior that gives you a wanted or unwanted outcome. Let's say you're thinking about applying for a job, for example, but you think that maybe you're not good enough. Suddenly, you experience a load of self-doubt. The self-doubt causes you to be hesitant, to question yourself. Perhaps you may not even try for the position and hide in the background where you won't be seen, even though you don't necessarily like it there. You don't get the job and stay right where you are as a result of believing the thought that you're not good enough. Nothing changes and you feel worse for it.

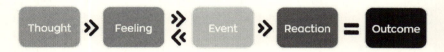

There are people who are driven by emotion. They feel their emotions first before noticing thoughts. A feeling triggers a thought about what's going on, which cues how you respond. Feeling self-doubt triggers a thought that you're not prepared for a final examination, which drives you to push yourself to study all night long. Cramming all night results in being utterly exhausted during and after the exam. The Thinking Habit Cascade helps the empathic person connect with their mind and the event to investigate what's going on inside to take back control.

The person closely tied to their emotions may notice their emotional weight by noticing their reaction or behavior triggered by their emotion. In this scenario, an emotion triggers a reaction then creates a thought about an event. Let's say you're feeling anxious. Anxiety triggers you to endlessly scroll through social media. While you're scrolling away you might be thinking that you can't handle everything that's going on at the moment. As a result, you're numbing away anxiety and putting off the things you want to do that's causing anxiety from not getting it squared away.

Likewise, a reaction can trigger a thought and feeling. Suppose you lash out at your husband for blocking the counter where you're preparing dinner. What feelings and thoughts are behind your behavior toward your husband? Perhaps you didn't get quality sleep because of restlessness. Feeling tired and wired, along with frustration, causes you to lash out. Your lashing out triggers negative thoughts about yourself after treating your husband unfairly and you lashing out at yourself for being unthoughtful.

The Thinking Habit Cascade is a simple, flexible, and elegant way to gain insight into what your brain is offering you to consider. This is the only mathematical type equation I have ever embraced and memorized. I remember the days of cramming as many physics, calculus, and chemistry formulas as possible on a 3" x 5" index card right before an exam. The Thinking Habit Cascades are much easier and highly applicable.

It's your choice whether you accept and attach onto any thought your brain offers. The choice is yours to remain in the negative space or to discover the freedom of stepping into the other side. The brain is doing its best with its antiquated system to make sense of our modern world. Engaging the logical prefrontal cortex is available, possible, and The Thinking Habit Cascade makes it doable.

The key to the model is knowing that a circumstance is an event; it's factual and specific as if you are submitting evidence to a court of law. Thoughts are the stories or sentences that we use to give meaning to the circumstance.

It's important to note that thoughts aren't always true or helpful, although the option to embrace a new way of thinking about a circumstance is always available to you. Don't be in a rush to change a thought because emotional processing needs to be done before moving forward. It's not necessarily a bad thing to hang in an unhelpful thought for a short bit. It's an opportunity to get to know it and discover what's lying underneath. That's how you begin to spotlight the shadowy thinking that can be cleaned up.

Feelings are bodily sensations. They're emotions. Emotions are energy created by biochemical reactions that move throughout the body. We tend to distract ourselves by reorganizing a kitchen drawer while a dreaded task waits to be completed, purchasing stuff you don't need, pouring another glass of wine because you've had a rough day, or helping yourself to another cupcake because we don't like to feel the discomfort. These are ways we cover up what we're feeling. The truth is that the human body is designed to process emotions. The sensations, although can be deeply uncomfortable, won't hurt, maim, or kill you. In fact, it's healthy to support your emotions to let them process, digest, and metabolize. Your massage therapist will thank you, for emotional metabolic waste can store in your muscles making them tight and painful. I'll walk you through emotional processing in Part III.

Reactions are how we behave in a situation, including what we don't do because of thoughts and feelings. Most people quit their new habit of eating 6 cups of equal proportions of dark and colorful greens, and sulfuric (onions, garlic, broccoli and cabbage) vegetables because they believe their brain when it says, "This is too much to eat," "Skipping a day or two won't change anything," or "I'm too tired to prepare all these vegetables." I hate to bust the proverbial bubble, but motivation and inspiration are created by your thoughts and feelings. Those thoughts and feelings are also blocking your ability to problem solve and brainstorm. They do not help you to make the problem better or to find ways to make eating 6 — 9 cups of vegetables daily possible. Folks don't take action because they're waiting for motivation to knock on the door. Motivation doesn't do that. You create it by choosing helpful thoughts that lead to a solution.

Every one of the cascades above gives you an outcome you are seeing in your life and health. That outcome is providing evidence to your brain that what it's thinking is true. A thought sets itself on repeat and soon it runs in the background without your awareness and becomes a thought habit. This is why unhelpful thinking can feel true to you.

The brain seeks patterns and associations and every bit of evidence it finds is determining your reality.

Taking a step back to examine what is happening in that beautiful head of yours can right the course at any time. Do you have a specific positive outcome in mind? Like resolving chronic fatigue by chance? Consider what thoughts and feelings you need to shift your behavior to one that is necessary to heal. Instead of entertaining self-pitying thoughts, choose to believe that you can figure out how to heal, which inspires research and trying new approaches that, in turn, push healing further into the recovery or highly manageable zone.

The Thinking Habit Cascade system of examining your problems offers an opportunity to objectively see what's happening and to create solutions to solving anxiety, worry, overwhelm, anger, fear, and doubt, by getting us to step out of our own way. It's an elegant yet powerful tool that gives the best possible outcome to anyone who steadily practices it by becoming a Thought Watcher observing their brain.

My thoughts are as quiet as me at times, which makes me an amazing observer of animals and people. On Friday nights, back in my high school days my best friend and I would watch travellers wordlessly go by at the airport. We made up stories about where folks were going while munching on fries from the café. Hearing my thoughts took practice to hear the words my mind quietly formed. Meditating and journaling helped me to slow down enough to actually hear.

Like myself, I noticed many of my clients are more prone to noticing feelings than thoughts. Instead of diving into the thinking, we begin by exploring emotions to then dig out the thoughts. There are also people who hear their thoughts more than their bodily sensations. For them we explore the thoughts while connecting back to the emotional body. There are others who don't notice their brain or body. We root around to see which way their system wants to work — body to brain or brain to body. We're all beautifully different. The elegance of the Thinking Habit Cascades offers the flexibility to examine the mind and body from a variety of angles.

EXAMINING YOUR THINKING HABITS

The first step in examining your mindset is to empty out your brain onto a piece of paper. In the last section I introduced and recommended starting a journaling practice. The power of healing through journaling is well known throughout psychology. Don't be afraid to put pen to paper and write it all out. If you're worried about privacy then create a secret hiding place for your journal, carry it with you at all times, or create a ritual to burn, bury, or release your written words by shredding when you decide it's time.

Start out by doing a brain dump for a few minutes. No need to spend hours journaling, unless that's truly your thing. 3-10 minutes is all you really need. Oftentimes I ask an open-ended question, such as "how do I feel today?" or "why am I upset when my spouse/co-worker/friend says or does [specifically what did they say or do]?" or I just free write whatever comes to mind. Bulleted lists, short sentences are all ok. There is no right or wrong way to empty what is running rampant in the mind.

What story are you telling yourself about what's happening? What are you making that mean? What are you making it mean about you?

Pull out those sentences or bulleted items that have a "need," "should," "have," "I am," or anything that is subjective. These are all your thoughts, my friend. This is a story forming with the intention of making meaning to what's causing those thoughts. Circle, highlight, or underline. Then choose the one that's most intriguing to you and let's put a magnifying glass to it.

FOREWARNING

Have you ever noticed that your immediate thought goes to "uh oh, what did I do now" or "she or he doesn't like me" or "they're out to get me" when a colleague, friend or family member wants to talk to you, offer feedback, or simply says something untowardly?

What about when you review a paper you've written or project completed? I'll bet you first focused on all the things wrong with what you've written or produced. Right?

The human brain automatically shifts to the negative. This negative bias is a mechanism meant to protect you from the wildlife stalking and ready to take you down for dinner. Don't be surprised when all the negativity bleeds onto your journal page. Most of all, don't avoid it either. Forward momentum doesn't take hold when the elephant in the room stays hidden. Tackling and healing that elephant turns it into a cuddly, snuggly chinchilla.

You may also notice that you believe one thing but react in total opposition to that belief, which is called cognitive dissonance. You can be motivated to write a couple of book chapters but find yourself mindlessly scrolling through Facebook. Or you choose to eat sugary treats when you know that sugar increases inflammation and pain in your body. These reactions typically manifest as anxiety, shame, regret, humiliation, unworthiness, and embarrassment.

A client of mine was struggling with adding movement to her daily routine. She truly believed that exercising daily would help her out of the sofa slump. During one of our sessions she expressed the frustration she had with herself about not doing her exercise. We discovered that her brain and body were in a tug of war over what type of movement each preferred. My client's belief about exercising daily meant she had to break a serious sweat pumping iron or running hard and fast around the neighborhood, like she used to. The more we explored she found that her body wanted gentle movement. She tried a variety of gentle movement exercise methods until she landed on Qi Qong, which is a gentle meditative practice that connects the brain and body. What's interesting to note is that Marie had always tackled everything she did with a lot of effort, which also contributed to accelerating her chronic fatigue cycle.

Negative bias and cognitive dissonance are normal! What's important is to become aware. Once you're aware then you have the opportunity to make better choices and changes.

What we think and believe matters. What you're thinking can disrupt the nervous system's healing state and deplete energy.

Viruses, bacteria, toxic mold, and hormones can send the brain into a thought-making tizzy. Simply knowing this possibility invites the opportunity to give yourself the grace and space to not react.

Managing thinking habits is doable but is only one piece of the holistic landscape to resolve chronic fatigue. Learning to work with your emotions is another vital habit to establish.

Repetitive thinking becomes unconscious and runs behind the scenes without our awareness. An unhelpful thought becomes an energy depleting habit.

Circumstances are things we cannot control, no matter how much we try. They're specific events no one can deny that triggers thoughts. Thoughts are sentences the brain makes up that in turn create emotions. Your feelings drive how you react. This entire cascade lands a result that provides evidence to your brain and you that whatever your thinking is true, even though the thought is probably not.

Regular downloading and examining of thoughts with the Thought Habit Cascade create an awareness of negative thinking habits that may be interrupting your healing. Once you see your thoughts, you then have the option to keep or let them go.

PUTTING THE THINKING HABITS CASCADE INTO ACTION

Examining your thoughts offers an opportunity to become acquainted with thinking patterns that are holding you back or keeping you stuck.

To examine your thinking, grab a piece of paper and pen and review the Thinking Habits Cascades. Write down everything on your mind about a specific event (a situation that's factual). Then plug in one of your thoughts, feelings, and reactions into any one of the five cascades to discover how your thought, feeling, and behavior habits are helping or not helping the situation.

Here are a few examples to get you started.

Examples:

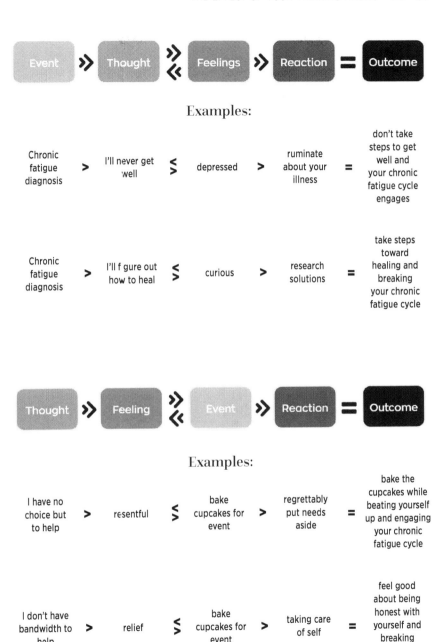

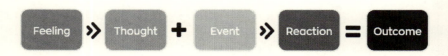

Examples:

| Restless | > | I need to get X done | + | get rest | > | tossing & turning & making list in your mind | = | no rest and chronic fatigue cycle engages |

| Calm | > | planning conserves my energy | + | get rest | > | plan your day/week with plenty of space for changes and rest | = | peacefully rest knowing you can easily pick up where you left off and breaking your chronic fatigue cycle |

Examples:

| Anxiety | > | eat a full pint of ice cream | > | I need to make today better + tough day | + | tough day | = | anxiety temporarily reduced, feel bloated, and chronic fatigue cycle engages |

| Compassion | > | meditate, take hot bath, read, and nap | > | What does my body need right now? | + | anxiety | = | Compassionate self-care that breaks your chronic fatigue cycle |

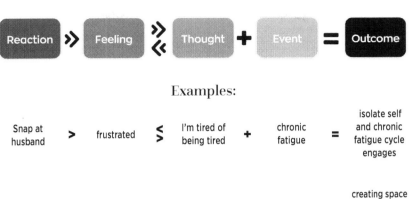

Examples:

Reaction		Feeling		Thought		Event		Outcome
Snap at husband	>	frustrated	<	I'm tired of being tired	+	chronic fatigue	=	isolate self and chronic fatigue cycle engages
Hands over heart	>	self-compassion	<	I need a moment to reconnect	+	frustration	=	creating space to consider what next step to take or what you need at the moment while breaking your chronic fatigue cycle

Seven

Food Habits: The Mind & Gut Connection

I mentioned earlier in this book that untended emotions often lead to health issues. Stomach pains and issues plagued me when I was younger. Now I see that anxiety and shame induced childhood experiences exacerbated future adulthood health issues. My first marriage was filled with anxiety and worry. Digestive issues began shortly after we married that worsened toward the end of our relationship. It's not fun asking your husband or friend to quickly pull over to go to the bathroom.

Digestive issues don't care about your schedule or location. Sitting in the middle seat of an airplane I was full of excitement to visit New Orleans for the first time. The flight had been uneventful with smooth sailing and quiet seat mates. I finished reading the magazine I picked up at the airport gift shop when the flight attendant announced that it was time to prepare for landing. There were about 15 minutes left before landing and before I could head toward the French Quarter to meet up with friends. Easing back, I closed my eyes, took a deep inhale when the gurgle made itself known. The plane was in its final descent, preventing my use of the lavatory, without having to make a scene.

Breathing deeply while wishing the gurgle away, the pressure made itself known more strongly. Quickly opening my eyes, I stared out the window willing the runway to show up RIGHT NOW! My legs bounced as I did my best to relax and breathe. The intestinal pressure continually built while I was petrified that an explosion was about to take place.

Immediately as the plane stopped at the jetway I bolted out of my seat, climbing over my aisle mate and pawing my way through the standing crowd as if an angry pack of dogs were chasing me. Somehow, I managed to make it just in time — *hallelujah!* Exiting the lavatory, I noticed the flight crew and, I swear, every single passenger was staring and laughing at me. This unfortunate scenario was my turning point.

Any situation where you find yourself assessing and strategically planning where bathrooms are is often a turning point for most to finally seek medical attention. Especially after one has such a public moment. There are numerous reasons why you're experiencing such urgency at the most inopportune times. I encourage you to feel the embarrassment and speak up to your physician. Be detailed with frequency and if you've noticed any type of pattern with foods or emotional upsets that trigger a flare.

Some conventional physicians may want to give you medications or offer advice to take Imodium and love your belly, especially if they don't find a specific cause for your distressed digestive system. After my gastroenterologist told me I needed to love my belly, I put my researching ways into finding an alternative medical resource.

I want to be clear that I am not dissing the physicians who devote themselves to learning medicine. Not in the least. Some physicians and specialists are generalists or get mired in the details of medical administration that the full connection between body and mind isn't seen. Additionally, conventional physicians have the additional burden of following medical insurance guidelines and rules. It's easy to see why it seems the human body has been compartmentalized to the point that the larger picture is no longer seen.

Conventional physicians are trained to treat symptoms and physical trauma, not to look deeper for a root cause. However, there are many conventional physicians that specialize in specific disorders, such as oncologists, rheumatologists, etc. Functional physicians treat illnesses using their foundation in conventional medicine and specialized training in functional medicine principles. Functional medicine principles look for the root cause of illness and offer treatments to resolve or significantly reduce symptoms using traditional and/or natural medicines. Some functional physicians, but not all, incorporate the principles of naturopathic medicine, which are based on treating a patient with natural or complementary treatment methods. If you're feeling less than satisfied with your health care team, your Inner Wisdom may be sending you a signal to dig deeper. Go to www.sharonwirant.com/tiredyetwired to find a list of resources, including directories for alternative medical practitioners.

Unfortunately, I was not having success with conventional medicine in my small town. I went from my primary physician to a gastroenterologist to a rheumatologist who enthusiastically announced that my "problem" explained my gut, body pain, and migraine issues. The rheumatologist was definitely correct that my health issues are all related, but his diagnosis of enteropathic rheumatoid arthritis meant prednisone and a heavy-duty drug with a side effect of cancer, which freaked me out. No diet change was recommended at all. Simply, take this pill once a day and you'll be ok. Yet, I wasn't.

My fitness instructor suggested seeking the help of a Functional Physician and reading the book, *The UltraMind Solution*, written by Dr. Mark Hyman. One of her clients had similar symptoms, found the book helpful, and was on her way to recovery working with a Functional Physician. This book made such an impact on me that I worked with Dr. Hyman's UltraWellness Clinic in Lenox, Massachusetts and later studied at the Institute of Integrative Nutrition to earn my health coach certification.

The Functional Physician is one who has an M.D. (Medical Doctor doctorate) and who wants to help patients from a deep level. They're determined to find the root cause using curiosity and critical thinking skills to learn our bodily systems and to be as precise as possible. There are Functional Physicians who specialize in specific conditions, such as hormones, sleep, autoimmune diseases, chronic fatigue, Lyme disease, or mold toxicity to name a few.

There are also the Naturopathic Physicians who also focus on solving the root cause and treat using natural methods. Like Functional Physicians, they use natural, herbal, and prescription medicines to help resolve or at least make manageable your medical concerns. There is a plethora of health care practitioners that specialize in chronic fatigue, adrenal fatigue, hormone balancing, Lyme disease, and mold toxicity.

I encourage you to research to locate resources near you. Check with your health insurance carrier about what they do and do not cover. Some insurances cover office visits and FDA approved testing only. Many Functional and Naturopathic Physicians don't handle insurance claims so be prepared to do the paperwork.

If you're telling yourself that you don't have a choice, that you have to stick with the physician you don't like, or there aren't alternative options then I suggest you question your thinking. When you're telling yourself there's no choice, you feel resigned and defeated. You quit, give in, succumb, and take no further action when you feel defeated. And you don't get better. You don't get better because you've given up.

MIND + GUT CONNECTION

Gastrointestinal discomfort — like bloating, cramping, gas, loose stool, urgent diarrhea — is an indicator of a possible problem in your gut. The lining of your gut loosens from exposure of a lot of the processed foods you ingest. Leaky gut, which this is called, not only causes digestive distress but also plays a role in your achy and stiff body, headaches, brain fog, and fatigue.

The loose gut lining lets in toxins that normally pass through and out. Your immune system goes to work as these toxins pass into other parts of your body that create a cytokine storm that leaves you feeling like you have the flu, body aches, inflammation, and brain fog. For some, a leaky gut causes weight loss and, for others, weight gain.

The effects of a leaky gut overworks the nervous system, negatively impacts the immune system, and encourages viruses, bacteria, and toxic mold to take up residence in your body.

What you invite into your body matters. Processed foods are manufactured to taste good and trigger dopamine, the "feel good" neurotransmitter. There's little nutritional value, which means you're creating quick burning energy rather than the slow burning sustainable energy that works best. Injecting yourself with energy by consuming caffeine and sugar-laden snacks and infused drinks quickly burns off or stores itself as fat while you end up tired, hungry, and overweight.

Consuming faux energy producing foods isn't doing your body a favor. A diet mostly consisting of carbohydrates and sugar produces glucose, which in turn is either quickly burned or stored as fat. My diet, which I thought was pretty darn healthy, prior to my leaky gut intervention consisted mostly of white flour and sugar products, sugar laden smoothies and juices, creamy pasta, and sandwiches because I was on the go and they were quick to prepare or purchase. My blood sugar level was all over the place. "Hangry," the act of being so hungry that you become impatient and likely to snap at someone, was an understatement with frequent sugar crashes and migraines.

I went cold turkey and dropped gluten, sugar, and dairy from my diet. I was determined. Not everyone can do that. To me, this diet was the way out of the anxiety and humiliation that goes with urgent GI distress. Again, the researcher in me delved into books and the internet to find recipes that matched approved foods for my condition, which have served me well over the last decade. I no longer take medication for migraines, rarely experience bloating, and my blood sugar levels are steady. I feel satiated that I no longer overeat, and generally feel energetic. More recently, I slightly adjusted my diet to help stymie mold toxicity. To be honest, I prefer and love eating fresh whole foods that make me feel energized and healthy.

The bottom line is that what we feed our bodies is either energy generating or depleting.

FOOD HABITS

Hippocrates said, *"Let food be thy medicine, and let medicine be thy food."* Food is medicine. What we eat influences our energy and state of health.

Throughout this book I am inviting you to think about what you are inviting into your body, mind and heart because what we focus on, we create. If you prefer tasty Doritos over a fresh green salad, then you're inviting in a quick fix of energy with little nutrition. Choosing a meal made with fresh vegetables with a side of lean protein means you're inviting in usable, nutritionally dense, and sustainable energy. A true healthy diet is one that's mostly vegetables, small portions of whole grains versus refined grains, and lean, pasture-raised meats, and sustainably caught fish. Dairy and sugar make up very little of a healthy diet. Sugar, including dairy, is an inflammatory food that makes autoimmune and chronic fatigue conditions worse. What you feed your body will either help or hinder your recovery from chronic fatigue.

A fresh whole food diet is best for the human species. A lot of greens and vegetables, a little whole grain (if you can tolerate), and a little lean protein are perfect. Be aware that most green juices and smoothies are full of quick burning sugar. Adding dark leafy greens with protein for breakfast, lunch, and dinner and you'll be satisfied while supporting your body down at the cellular level to produce quality energy.

Do your body a favor by leaving refined sugar behind. Once you start reading ingredient labels on food you'll be surprised at how much sugar most pre-packaged foods contain. The best sugars to eat are directly from whole fruits and berries. Instead of using refined white sugar in baked goods, consider using dates, coconut nectar, or coconut sugar, or none at all. I invite you to a 30-day sugar elimination trial. I guarantee you'll feel better without the sugar. Now that I've eliminated refined sugar from my diet, I can't even eat most store bought treats because they're sickeningly sweet.

Cheese is another inflammatory culprit that needs to be eliminated or eaten only as an occasional treat. It was surprising to learn that cheese acts like sugar in that it's fast burning and stores glucose in fat.

Cheese also increases mucus production and a histamine response. My sinus congestion, runny nose, and throat clearing practically disappeared when I stopped eating cheese. In all honesty, sugar was easier for me to eliminate but I had a hard time resisting cheese. I've finally knocked that food habit, and my ability to breathe has gotten so much better.

What I hear the most as a coach is that clients "don't have time," "there's no way I can eat 6 or more cups of veggies a day," "that type of food is bland," and "cooking is a chore." These are all thoughts preventing you from creating energy from the inside. When you tell yourself these types of things then you don't consider trying a new recipe, figuring out how to spice up the flavors with herbs, and preparing meals in advance.

- What if preparing meal plans and meals ahead of time is actually saving you time?
- What if fresh herbs improve the flavors of your meal and offer you extra benefits?
- How do you feel when you eat food off your plan?
- How do you feel when you do eat food on your plan?
- What's the cost of you eating food off your plan?
- What is the benefit of eating foods on your plan?

MINDFUL EATING

Life is busy. Meals are eaten quickly to move on to the next thing. Slowing down while eating gives you an opportunity to enjoy foods. Ready-to-go and processed foods make it so easy to grab a handful of chips and down a soda because you're starving. Savoring food offers an opportunity to discover what foods feel great and not so great in the body.

Try Mindful Eating. Mindful Eating is about taking a bite of food, setting down your fork or spoon, and chewing your food slowly while you take in the flavors and textures.

Here's the exercise in detail: sit down with your meal in front of you. Take 3-5 slow and full breaths. Pick up your fork and eat a small forkful of a piece of food. Set down your fork. Chew your food 20 — 40 times. Breathe while you are chewing slowly. Notice how the food tastes and feels in your mouth. Swallow. Continue breathing as the food settles in your belly. Sit and breathe for several more breaths. Notice how your body feels as it begins to digest the food you offered it. Take note of how your body feels as you eat and digest.

Eating mindfully has shaped my food nourishment plan. There are many different types of food lifestyle choices — Autoimmune Protocol (AIP), Whole30, Low Mold, Keto, Mediterranean, and Paleo to name a few. I've chosen a Paleo type diet, which is heavy vegetable, complex carbohydrates (sweet potatoes vs white potatoes), pasture-raised meats, no grains, no dairy, and no sugar as my choice of food lifestyle. I then made adjustments to support a low mold diet by eliminating a few food items like mushrooms and vinegar. For me, my compelling reason to stick to the diet I chose is how good I feel. Being mindful of what I put into my body feels refreshing from the inside out. Eating off my plan, I feel terrible, and my GI system is unhappy. My joints feel inflamed and achy while my belly feels like a chunk of lead sitting in the pit of my stomach. Which do I prefer to feel? The light, refreshing, and satisfied version of me for sure!

There is no one particular diet that I recommend nor is it the scope of this book to detail each food lifestyle option. Your best bet is by following what your body needs in light of what is contributing to your chronic fatigue, any autoimmune conditions, and what feels good in your body. Start by changing one thing at a time and allow yourself some grace when you slip up. Tomorrow is always a great day to start again. I highly suggest working with a knowledgeable and qualified nutritionist who understands your health needs. Head over to www.sharonwirant.com/tiredyetwired to find a directory to locate a qualified nutritionist nearest you.

One thing you may notice when you switch to a whole foods diet or autoimmune supportive diet is that you'll feel satiated and lose weight, especially when you combine doing the thought and emotional work I discuss in upcoming chapters.

BODY DETOX

Supporting your body with detoxing all the toxins accumulated from a poor nutrition diet is also essential. This is actually my favorite body support act! Detox is not about deprivation. Detoxing is about toxin elimination while filling yourself with nourishment. While I love cooking and flavorful healthy foods, a long Epsom salt bath with fragrant lavender oil and a good book with soft music in the background is one of my favorite ways to de-stress. My body holds onto emotions and energy from outside of me (as well as inside of me) and water dispels all that excess depleting energy.

Dry brushing before showering sloughs off old skin cells and stimulates lymph drainage. Your skin can breathe and release toxins. Use a natural brush, like sisal, with moderately stiff bristles. Starting at your feet brush upwards toward your heart. Don't forget to brush your back, too. Then hop into a nice, warm shower or bath.

At the end of every shower, I significantly drop the temperature as I rinse my hair and twirl for another rinse or two in the shower. Deciding to embrace my Nordic roots by getting hot and sweaty then chilling off boosts my immune system.

Sweating encourages toxins out of the body. Be sure to work up a good sweat through movement, hot Epsom salt baths, or regularly take a sauna. I move every day, whether that's Pilates, yoga, or a hike with the dogs. I move with purpose to get the inside of the flow of my body. Recently, we purchased a low EMF infrared sauna, which is amazing. Sweating up a storm leaves me feeling refreshed and my skin looking healthy. I've had my best sleep since implementing a regular sauna routine yet. While sitting in my Easy Bake™ oven, I imagine mycotoxins exiting through the sweat streaming out of my body. While not everyone has room for an in-home sauna, there are a variety of options to get your sweat on. Your local gym or health club may have available saunas, you may borrow a friend's sauna, or you can put money aside to purchase a personal sauna. There are many inexpensive sauna options ranging from blankets to portable huts to small closet-sized boxes. Start setting aside the money you'd spend on

Starbucks drinks, which contain too much inflammatory sugar and dairy, to purchase a sauna if that lights you up.

Over the years, I have always said that our home is a resort minus the staff. We've created healthy and inspiring spaces in our home — a Pilates/yoga/meditation space in the loft, a "She Studio" creative space, a hot tub, sauna, gorgeous mountain views, and hiking trails just a step outside the house. Our living spaces display items that spark joy — my mother's art, books, trinkets from my deceased grandparents, and pictures of loved ones. We keep only what we enjoy while reducing clutter and making upkeep quick and easy. Plants fill the sunny Great Room to provide fresh clean air and a touch of indoor nature. Air purifiers boost air cleanliness and freshness in each room of our home. Scented candles and essential oil aromatherapy are often lit to help our body and mind relax and discourage bacteria, virus, and mycotoxins from our inner and outer spaces. See — what you *think* you really do *create*!

Movement is important to get your blood flowing, which delivers oxygen and nutrients to cells throughout your body and to eliminate more toxins. When you begin a movement plan, especially if you're just starting out, be sure that you pay close attention to what your body is telling you even while you're moving. It's easy to push through and do more than your body is ready for. I was a champion in this category.

Taking a hike in nature has always been a priority even when I was frequently traveling. Some destinations had easily accessible parks and trails but just as many were in the middle of nowhere so the hotel gym treadmill or yoga in my room were my best options. I always made time for even just 15 minutes. The sicker I became the more exercise hurt afterwards. A short hike on a trail left me in a lot of pain and stiffness and I wouldn't exercise for days and weeks afterwards. Weekends where I ran with my dogs for 60 seconds up to 18 times each day left me hurting badly, popping Motrin like candy and pumping up my attitude to push through to keep on going. Continually pushing myself physically clearly contributed to my collapse.

Weekend warriors give their all throughout the work week then pump it up a few notches over the weekend under the guise of self-care as a form of play. Play can turn into more work, another expectation, and sneakily energy depleting. Spending every free moment either training, attending workshops, or competing at dog agility trials, I wore myself out. I wore out because of a heavy travel load for work then headed out to long weekend competitions. Competing entailed packing up us and the dogs then driving to the trial site. We'd arrive late, set up, grab a light dinner then head to bed. Early morning wake-up calls, poor quality sleep, a full slate of classes, lots of socializing, and rarely sitting down for a break set me up for an adrenal burnout while cranking up the chronic fatigue cycle.

You can accomplish anything if you push yourself hard enough but what's the cost? Yes, I had a dream job and lots of accolades, trophies, and ribbons acknowledging my skill and knowledge. The cost of ignoring my body's pleas for rest resulted in years of having to rest. I resisted rest because then I was faced with all the physical and emotional discomfort I felt inside. Like many humans, I numbed my pain and wounds by keeping busy.

My hobby had turned into yet another job depleting me of energy. I'm far from ready to give up the game but my inner work is all about how I experience and participate in competitions in the future. What depletes me? Energizes me? Why do I want to attend this trial? Why do I not want to attend this trial? What do I want to experience? And, how can I make that experience happen? These are great questions to ponder if you, too, engage in a hobby that seems to have taken over your life.

Working with a chronic fatigue, Lyme, mold, or autoimmune-literate physician is your first course of action. Know what you are dealing with then start applying a medical and food treatment plan. Medication and food support your body to start healing and generating energy.

Working with my healthcare team, all of whom specialize in hormones, fatigue, Lyme and mold, was the first and most important piece of my chronic fatigue puzzle to resolve. Without their knowledge, experience, and treatment plans I don't believe I'd be where I am today. They got me on the right path by treating me appropriately with medications you can't get off the counter. I supplemented their treatment with thought and emotional heart work. Thought work worked up to a point then I struggled until I was introduced to addressing my emotional wounds from the little challenging life events that I mentioned in Chapter 2. You don't always know what you're holding onto. What I needed was to connect with my body and heart to feel and heal.

We all have practiced unhelpful thoughts and untended wounds because we're not taught how nor are they even spoken about aloud. These are the shadows we hide in that stop us from stepping out or speaking up or doing what feels right. The shadows fuel the fire that is chronic fatigue. Let's shine a light on them by clearing the way and supporting our body with the medicine, nutrition, and movement it needs and craves then weeding the garden from the toxic weeds preventing the growth of the beautiful bloom that's you.

Your first step in energy generation is to take your medications, begin fueling your body with fresh foods, start moving and sweating then give attention to your mindset and emotions.

My role is to help clients first get their body started on the healing path by helping them stay on track by eliminating pathogens as directed from a healthcare practitioner and integrating a nutritional support plan prescribed by a nutritionist. Once your treatment and nutrition plan are set, we level up your healing path by managing your thinking and feeling your feelings. Those toxic, thick weeds that choke the healing path are what you're thinking and feeling (or not feeling). The next step to weeding the garden within you is to examine your mindset to know what beliefs you're holding onto that block your flower from blooming. Once you become aware of those thoughts and beliefs, you have the choice and ability to choose new beliefs and create the change you're craving.

Those sugary delights and caffeinated drinks paired with overthinking, an ultra busy lifestyle, and numbing out any uncomfortable feeling are the ingredients that are making you tired yet wired. Your body is tired but can't rest because the fuel you're offering and the lightning fast pace you're trying to keep up with is running on automatic. Your brain, your emotions, and your body are all running at the same time, like a pilot light ready to ignite a fire at any moment.

Now that you've learned about the impact of nutrition, behavior habits, thinking habits, emotional habits, and their effect on your immune system, let's turn that tired yet wired feeling into one that is calm, peaceful, relaxed, and at ease by cultivating a resilient body, mind, heart, and soul.

PART III

Reset + Reconnect + Recover

CULTIVATING A RESILIENT BODY, MIND, HEART, & SOUL

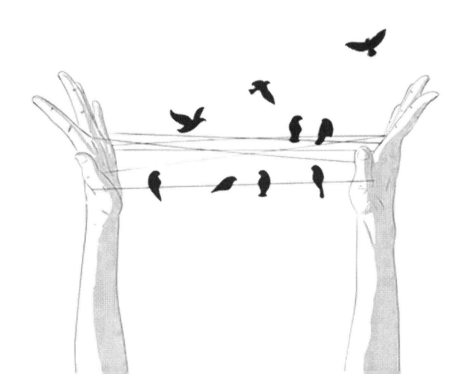

Eight

Tending to the Garden of You

Stepping inside the big glass castle looking building of the local Conservatory and Botanical Garden I'm hit with the fresh fragrance and humidity of clean, nourishing earth. The space inside is silent yet I can hear the soft whispers of the plants within. If I'm lucky enough I may catch sight of a butterfly or other pollinating insect buzzing around looking for a sip of nectar. For hours I wander around taking in the sights, smells, colors, and textures of each, and every plant within this glass building. The energy within feels calm, soothing, and very relaxing. The Botanical Garden is the perfect spot to do a little deep thinking, sketching, or gazing in awe at the flora surrounding me. The serene and tranquil vibe of the botanical garden is how I've always wanted to feel.

    Botanic gardens and conservatories are peaceful and beautiful spaces to visit, especially when many of the plants are in full glorious bloom. Master Gardeners tend to the needs of plants every day, no matter what. They uproot unhelpful weeds, trim unruly branches and shoots, and keep the soil properly hydrated. Shoots and thinned-out bulbs are propagated then transplanted to bring life to more botanical species. Pollen from flowers is collected and spread to other flowers to ensure future varieties and blossoms can be enjoyed and nourish the bees. Each plant is lovingly cared for by the gardening caretakers. Tending to the body, mind, heart, and soul gives one a sense of aliveness laced with calmness.

Likewise, caregivers in any industry ensure that those under their care have all their needs taken care of — food, water, warmth, shelter, and a shoulder to lean on — usually ahead of or in lieu of their own. Prioritizing others ahead of yourself, without a self-care plan in place, is physically, emotionally, mentally, and energetically depleting for you, the owner of your body. The misprioritization insists your nervous system to keep on protecting. Amplification of the nervous system needs to be slowed down to generate a calm aliveness that resides within our internal environment.

The garden of you consists of your physical body, mind, heart, and soul. All these components are entwined. They work in synchrony yet also individually. The exquisite complexity of human nature often clogs up the works when one system isn't running at full efficiency. Tending to the needs of our body, mind, emotions will nurture your entire being into a beautiful, healthy version of you. To live life as the best version of you.

It seems that our culture frowns upon prioritizing self-care. There are unspoken messages that our spouse, children, friends, and employers come well before ourselves. Self-care is often seen as frivolous, too luxurious, and only for those with money. This is one big fat lie. Your crystal flute filled with a sparkly expensive French champagne isn't full enough for you to enjoy the fine, crisp, sparkly elixir when you put yourself at the bottom of the list. Instead, there's only a mere drop or two of liquid gold on the bottom for your enjoyment.

Self-care is also not simply about drinking green smoothies, spa treatments, manicures, pedicures, massages, and bubble baths. These delights are certainly selections to include in your personal care tending basket, though aren't the only items on the self-care menu to choose from.

This section is about tending to the garden of you by activating a nourishing and healing body, mind, heart, and soul. Self-care is like the Master Gardener tending to a luscious garden so that it flourishes, thrives, grows, and blooms to its full beautiful, fragrant, and colorful potential. Healing from chronic fatigue requires self-care. There is no magic pill that will eliminate your symptoms with a quick nod of the head and twitch of the nose like Tabitha of *Bewitched*. Medications, supplements, and herbal treatments are effective treatments, but they can't heal what you're thinking and feeling inside. Tending to your thoughts and feelings is key to a healthy and thriving life.

My client, Sarah, came to me on the suggestion of her physician. She was on the right medical treatment plan but struggled with chronic fatigue and frequent crashes. She had caught the usual virus going around her office, but unlike her co-workers, she never bounced back. With me she learned tools to help her slow the onslaught of thoughts to calm her nervous system. Through our coaching sessions and creating her own timeline, her illness struck shortly after having a stressful challenging life situation. While she loved her chosen line of work, she never expected to be caught in the middle of a serious workplace incident that resulted in a firing of an employee. The employee that got fired was a close friend, who she often went shopping with and to lunch with on a regular basis. Under any normal circumstance, being involved in a firing wasn't a big deal. Letting employees go was part of her work responsibilities as a human resource professional, but the stress of being involved in this specific incident resulted in the loss of a friendship that carried a deep sense of guilt and shame. In addition, this scenario reflected a deep reminder about her parents contentious divorce when she was 8 years old. While her behavior habit of working a lot, helping her family and volunteering in the community, as well as a dwindling marriage, this recent event probably ignited her chronic fatigue cycle. She was stressed, giving more to others than herself and grieving a friendship. She fought the emotions within her as she attempted to keep herself together until becoming so ill that a medical leave of absence was necessary. Digging further into her behavior, thoughts, and emotional habits, we put a spotlight on those patterns she wanted to break with and that kept her feeling small and hidden. Seeing the effects of her unhelpful thoughts and feelings, she could choose a new direction with understanding.

Together we explored and adjusted her thinking, behavior habits, and being with and understanding the emotions causing her crashes and fatigue. She learned to accept and support herself first, turn the volume down on her Inner Critics, befriend and listen to her feelings, and align with her true self. Sarah began taking care of herself with tools I offer in this book, along with many coaching techniques to create breakthroughs. By creating her personalized care tending basket, she now has tools and resources at a moment's notice to halt the chronic fatigue cycle. Nowadays, her crashes are infrequent and usually in response to ignoring the early signals telling her to back off. She's back at her job, has gradually worked up to a full-time schedule, and feels happy, content, and energetic. She's returned to helping others and volunteering if she wants rather than because she has to, and started reconnecting in her marriage.

Like Sarah, taking care to cleanse my mind of unnecessary lies, befriending both my Inner Rebel and Inner Critic, and embracing emotions that flow led to becoming a confident and fierce advocate for myself. Doing inner work helps you to make decisions and choices from a clean place that offers freedom rather than the emotional pain of victimhood. In turn, I let go of those who teased and implied self-care is only for the weak and took back my power by listening to what my body, heart, and soul wants. There is only one life as far as I know. I am determined to enjoy and live a life that fulfills me rather than what someone else thinks it should be.

No one knows what you need more than you. Learning to have your own back while knowing exactly how to take care of yourself is where the magic lies. Expectations and blaming others for not providing what we need is not productive nor sustainable. Whole-heartedly accepting the responsibility of your own thoughts, feelings, and actions brings about the peace, ease, and calm your body needs to heal. As a bonus, a spaciousness to love, give, and receive grows larger and stronger than before.

The way to break the spell of chronic fatigue is to fully care for you — body, mind, heart, and soul — by cleansing your mindset and tending to those wounds by feeling the feels. Stepping into the courage to shine a bright spotlight onto the shadows within you offers the freedom to live life on your terms and to take back your precious energy. Shining that light gives you the opportunity to discover and redesign what were once limitations. Exposing and changing those limitations invites your body to heal with energy to spare.

I can't encourage you enough to begin a daily practice to help guide your day the way you intended. Apply the tools and exercises I'm sharing with you. Doing the inside work is where your freedom from fatigue lies. The more you try and apply, the better you will begin to feel.

Get out of your head and into your body. Become aware of all the thoughts running in your head then selectively choose the ones to keep and ignore the others. This takes practice and permission from you to allow yourself grace when you don't catch a thought or wallow in an emotion. It will happen because you are beautifully human. Put any self-judgment and criticism on a shelf and give yourself a little hug whenever a mistake happens.

Do your best to let go of what you resist. Because what you resist loves to persist.

Growth requires change and change requires commitment to do the work.

You have choices with anything you think, feel, or do. You can choose to implement lifestyle changes if you want to heal and recover. Getting back to your regular activities is a possibility by paying attention, closely monitoring, and refilling your energy tank well before it gets depleted. Ideally, you want to plan on keeping your tank overfilled and spending energy from the spillage. There will be major changes in your life — diet change, a regular meditation and gentle exercise practice, new social community, and a slower paced life.

Or you can decide to stay where you are with continued exhaustion, frequent and intense crashes, and not living the life you are dreaming about. That choice is yours.

If you're choosing to find yourself on the other side of chronic fatigue, then you're committing to do what it takes to get that result.

I choose to live deliberately, despite a life full of diagnosis after diagnosis. There are still many places I want to visit, relationships to strengthen and new ones to cultivate, to inhale the fresh ocean and mountain air, and to contribute to this wonderful world of ours while feeling energetic, clear, and at ease. My compelling reason to do whatever it takes to recover is because, to me, there is too much of life I don't want to miss, too much I have left to give, and too much I want to see.

As I began treatment, my daily mantra became, "I'm making my body hostile to pathogens." This affirmation reminded me daily why I wanted to heal. My goal of recovering didn't include only medications, supplements, and diet change. I looked at all areas of my life that were less than satisfactory because they were playing a major role. What did I want? Why was healing from chronic fatigue important to me? What I wanted required commitment — to say no, to slow down, to do things differently or I'd end up right back where I started as my history clearly predicts. My why is my commitment.

WHAT'S YOUR WHY & COMMITMENT

1. Grab a piece of paper or, better yet, start a new journal. On the first page write yourself a letter about why you want to tend the garden of you. Use the questions below to guide your letter:
   - What is your why? Why is healing from chronic fatigue important to you?
   - What is the cost of not committing or following through?
   - What are the possible benefits of doing this work?

2. Write out your why in one sentence on a couple of pieces of paper, post-it's, or note cards. Place these notes where you see them often — the mirror, closet door, nightstand, refrigerator, computer screen, or daily planner. Remind yourself why healing matters to you.

Nine

Cultivating a Thriving Mindset

You feel like what's happening in your head resembles the ping pong balls tossing about in the lottery bubble machine. Instead of grabbing the winning ping pong balls for a multi-million-dollar prize, you're feeling anxious, overwhelmed, and out of control. You feel your heart pounding away while your entire body is vibrating. Loud mental chatter and bodily sensations make you want to jump out of your skin. Creating more projects, keeping busy, and running here, there, and everywhere help dull that wired feeling.

I remember there would be days, especially after traveling, that being overwhelmed was mild compared to how overwhelmed I felt. Sitting at my desk, kitchen table, sofa, and even in bed my body and brain would freeze up as I reviewed my list of to-do's, reading emails, or articles. My thoughts were spinning so fast that I couldn't catch the words while my body hotly hummed like electricity through a wire. Between the whirling thoughts and my buzzing body, distraction was my antidote for avoidance. On top of avoiding work, sleep was not to be had at nighttime. Sleep came in about 90-minute increments while my mind spun on all the things I didn't get done and still needed to do. My mind would whirl and twirl until my body and brain finally gave up from exhaustion at 4 am.

Thoughts can be a scathing commentary of feedback, of what you've done wrong, what you need to edit, revise, or totally redo, a rundown on all your to-do's. There's too much to do with little available time, and your thoughts are holding a loud and rowdy pity party in your head. The body responds appropriately to your brain's declarations and bawdy singing.

All this brain activity is mentally (and physically) draining from the constant ping-ponging back and forth. The overwhelm and anxiety rises in your body because of this thought frenzy. The thoughts are coming faster than you can catch but you notice them. You feel them, too. The nervous system reacts to your brain and emotional messages and ramps up production of adrenaline, a fight or flight hormone that increases your heart and respiration rates, and boosts energy.

Tending to our minds is a necessity. The brain conjures up 50 to 60 thousand thoughts a day! It's busy trying to sort patterns and associations to decide what to keep or toss aside with its first line of defense to warn you of all the dangers. Remember, the mind is programmed toward a negative bias in an effort to keep us safe from the lions, tigers, and bears stalking and ready to pounce on us for their delicious meal of the day.

Most of us are wandering around letting our minds run wild and unleashed. We think that we can't control our thoughts and that they should just stop. The deal is that thoughts pop up whenever we attend to them. We aren't taught that we can choose what thoughts to keep and act on. The cool thing is that the thoughts we act on are the ones that pop up the most. What we can control is the impact of our thinking by being selective with the thoughts we decide to keep.

That was me. This "go with the flow" gal let her brain go off on amazing adventures and replay serious haunts. I clung to too many thoughts that weren't serving me well and, quite frankly, were not at all true, though my mind sought out evidence to convince me otherwise. But as I learned to dig deeper into the layers, I started to see how I was limiting myself by my very own thoughts.

STILLNESS

Stillness is getting in tune with yourself and nature. Your energy vibration of your overworking nervous system quiets down and begins to cool. Getting still connects our mind and body in a way that's nurturing and frees your intuition. Your senses awaken and you begin to notice your breathing, mind, and body. This connection is a key to freeing yourself from chronic fatigue and the many stressors in life. Before I could sort through all those racing thoughts, I needed to slow my brain down.

Meditation is all about getting still. For those with chronic fatigue, developing a meditation or stillness practice supports our nervous system, mind, and emotions.

Many people cannot sit or be still. The mind and body are too restless to settle enough to get still. I was one of them. Always needing to read a book, watch television, or scroll through social media, and the news outlets. Learning to sit and be is challenging but well worth the effort.

A form of meditation that I committed to in the beginning of my journey is a Native American meditation method called Sit Spot. I learned the Sit Spot meditation method from a mentor, Michael Trotta of *Sagefire Institute*. Sit Spot resonated with me because it's nature-based and I didn't have to sit on a pillow with my eyes closed chanting "*ohm*." Google Sit Spot meditation and you'll find lots of options.

Sit Spot meditation is about sitting outside in nature while using your five senses: visual, auditory, tactile, olfactory, and gustatory. Sitting in a quiet spot, you simply notice 3 to 4 different things you can see near, far, and in your periphery. Listen for 3 to 4 different loud and soft sounds. Feel different sensations on your body and skin. Pay attention to the different smells on the wind and nearby. And, lastly, see what you can taste in the air. You'd be surprised how nice fresh cut grass tastes. Once you notice all the sights, sounds, and sensations around you then settle in to be with what you feel on the outside and inside of you. Close your eyes, take everything in or, if you prefer, leave your eyes open and gaze softly onto the natural world.

Every day I sit or walk outside in stillness. My favorite spot is either the stone wall or a secret spot on our property when I don't want to be found. After taking several deep cleansing breaths I settle into my spot. I say a short intention and ask for wisdom for a solution. Continuing a slow yet full breathing pattern, I use my eyes to look near, far, and wide to notice 3 or 4 different things. Then I move on to the other senses — smell, tactile, auditory, and taste. I sit in my spot fully aware of what I'm seeing, hearing, smelling, feeling, and tasting as I allow thoughts to come and go and body sensations to flow in and out. Most of the time my eyes are kept open, but there are times I prefer to close my eyes to focus more closely as I settle into the stillness within and around me. As stillness settles in you may notice chipmunks, dragonflies, birds, or a fox step into your view or very close if not on you. What's happened is that you've lowered your energy frequency that indicates you're not a threat. This, my friends, is my favorite part.

Sit Spot meditation can be up leveled by taking your stillness for a walk in the forest. Being out in nature is good to reconnect, recenter, and reset your nervous system. Animal trackers use this skill of becoming still to locate animals on safari. Bird watchers and photographers use stillness to find that elusive bird or animal they've been searching for. Sitting in the back of a pickup truck in the middle of the Botswana savannah searching for birds with the "birders" of our group taught me the power of stillness. Each morning as our group selected which safari vehicle to ride in, I always hustled to the birder's truck. The birders meandered, paused, then meandered again. While my group mates were busy searching, identifying, and photographing birds, I kept my eyes on the ground to see what mammals might poke their heads up. I checked off many animals off my list that most of my groupmates didn't see because they were more intent on seeing the bigger animals, like elephants, lions, and giraffes.

Once I learned to get still the exploration and cleansing of my mind could begin.

QUICK START THOUGHT CONTROL

Thoughts that are racing, judgmental, and constantly worrying about worst-case scenarios can easily catch you off guard and build up anxiety and overwhelm. You may have meditated earlier in the day, but the thoughts became unruly again.

When you let those thoughts run rogue, anxiety can blow through the roof. The anxiety from an unmanaged mind shows up three different ways:

1. You might try to **fight** the anxiety by doing more, learning more, and frequently checking in with sources in the know.
2. Anxiety can find you **fleeing** to escape by numbing yourself, passively consuming online or in-person workshops, binging Netflix, submerging yourself in needless tasks, indulging in an extra cocktail or dessert each night, or perhaps buying lots of dog gear (like myself) or stuff you really don't need. You're simply trying to escape the discomfort of it all.
3. Lastly, anxiety can **stop** you in your tracks. Overwhelm keeps you plastered on the sofa. Depleted energy causes you to collapse with no capacity to get yourself up. All you want is to remain in the fetal position hidden far under the blankets.

These three scenarios bring about an awful lot of emotional suffering. It's okay to feel what you're feeling, but what we want to prevent is you going way down into the rabbit hole by ruminating on those thoughts.

How do you stop these thoughts from racing? If you aren't able to meditate, then here's a way to slow down the thoughts and come back to the present moment where you can then make adjustments to your thinking. Remember, you are not and don't have to be your thoughts.

Applying this simple exercise helps you recenter, reconnect, and refocus by calming your mind and resetting your nervous system into a more soothing, healing state. When your body is in a healing state you preserve your energy, stop the swirl of thoughts and anxiety to get back to the present moment and be intentional about what you want to do next.

Think about it, when our smartphones and computers get wonky the best solution, most of the time, is to turn it off, wait 30 seconds, and then turn it back on. We can do the same for ourselves by stopping, taking several deep breaths before moving forward.

C.A.L.M.R. is a 5-step process that gives you a reset button to release past and future thinking and to be calmly in the present instead of living in the freak out zone.

This exercise can be done in any position, sitting, standing, or even lying down. Be sure your feet are firmly on the floor if you're sitting or standing. My favorite place to do this exercise is outdoors in the fresh air and nature.

Throughout this exercise you'll use a simple breathing pattern: *slowly inhale through the nose* filling your belly and heart center/chest area, *slowly exhale through the mouth* making a soft sigh sound.

I recommend closing your eyes but leave them open if that feels best for you.

> **Step 1: Check in** — Pause to check in with yourself. Feel free to sit, stand, or lay down on a comfortable surface. Your eyes can be open or closed. Place your hands over your heart. Inhale/exhale 3x
>
> **Step 2: Accept & Interrupt** — Interrupt your overworking brain by lightly tapping your hand over your heart then hold your top hand out in a 'stop' gesture. Firmly yet gently say, "stop." No need to be harsh at all. You are supporting, NOT criticizing yourself. This action begins the reset of your mind and body into calmness.
>
> **Step 3: Lean In** — Lean into the moment. No judgments or analyses are to be made. Just be. Inhale in through your nose filling up your belly all the way up to your heart center with air. Exhale fully through your mouth. Continue this breathing pattern.
>
> **Step 4: Mindful** — Create awareness within. Shift your attention from your head to your bottom supported in the chair then your feet on the ground. Notice any

sensations but there's no need to name them, just notice them. Continue the breathing pattern, and focus on feeling your feet supported by the ground.

Step 5: Reset — Stay here as long as you like by continuing the breathing pattern and feeling yourself supported by the ground until you notice a shift into calmness, relaxation, a settling, or centeredness!

Thank yourself aloud — *well done, great job, thank you* — and give your arms a squeeze for doing this practice. When you're ready, gradually bring yourself back to the present moment. You're brain and body love when you acknowledge it.

Take time to reflect on your experience to find clarity of what thought and feeling patterns were speaking out.

This exercise can be used as often as you'd like. What I love most is that this exercise can be used on an as needed basis or as a preventative. To use this tool as a preventative, set a reminder on your phone every 2 to 3 hours to alert yourself to taking a pause to regroup. I highly recommend selecting a calming chime-type ringtone. An extra bonus is that after many repetitions, the calm and soothing ringtone automatically causes you to breathe and relax. C.A.L.M.R. gives your body a reset that ignites healing and you'll feel better in a short time.

You can find a video demonstration at: www.sharonwirant.com/tiredyetwired

THE THOUGHT CLEANSE

Now that you're starting to slow down, let's slow down all that mind chatter. It's time to catch thoughts. You have to know what you're thinking so you can decide which ones to keep and which to toss out the window. Every day take the time to slow down with a short meditation or a series of 3-6 or more deep full breaths then conduct a brain dump. Download everything on your mind. Grab a piece of paper or a favorite journal and purge all your thoughts. Allow yourself to be uncensored.

Oh, boy, I felt the resistance there! Many people don't want to know what their brain is actually saying. I get it because I didn't either. Approach your thought downloads with curiosity to see what's there. Knowing what's happening inside your mind is fascinating once you start listening on a regular basis. The best part is that once you know what your thinking habits are then you can change them to be of service for you and alter the course of your health and life.

Buy yourself a beautiful journal. One that you want to touch and see every day. Then every morning for 5-10 minutes, or whatever time slot works best for you, pull out your journal to write out everything that is on your mind. Know that you can brain dump or journal in the morning, evening, or whenever you feel anxiety, heaviness, overwhelm, or worry rears her pretty head. There is no set schedule but be sure that you actually do this part. Your brain is not a file cabinet. Keeping those unhelpful thoughts stored inside invites the brain to offer them to you time and time again.

For those of you who are worried that someone might read your entries or that you're hiding secrets, I invite you to question that thinking. You're more likely to censor your writing. What if putting your thoughts on paper is your safe place where you can reveal your vulnerabilities without the fear of being judged? I bet you're more likely to keep your journal handy in the event that you need a purge than to keep it under lock and key. I also had this worry in the beginning of my journaling journey. Instead of worrying, I decided that my journal is my around the clock therapist that I could talk to at any moment. Once I made the decision I was all in with this emptying my brain exercise. The lightness and clarity that comes from journaling is worth questioning the resistance.

You also don't need to be an eloquent writer or even grammatically correct. All you need is paper and pen to write down in any form what's on your mind. Write a bulleted list or single sentences. If you love to write, then consider writing 2-3 pages every day. There's no right or wrong way here, just get all those thoughts out of your head.

Do you prefer to put pen to paper or typing into your computer or tablet? Either way is totally acceptable. That's up to you but there's a ton of research supporting that writing with pen in hand is the most effective.

Ask yourself questions that inspire you to take action, create, or find a solution. Be sure that you ask a question that's explorative. I've listed a few below and you can download a list at www.sharonwirant.com/tiredyetwired. You can also find many journals specifically for this purpose online.

- What about this circumstance bothers me?
- What can I take away from this experience?
- What is going well in my life/relationships/work/health, etc.?
- What if this all works out?
- What do I want to do now?
- What does my body want or need?
- What do I want my day to look like?
- What do I want my relationship with [person] to look like?

Take a quick look at what you wrote. Here is where the Thinking Habit Cascades from Chapter 6 come into play. What is the problem, event, or incident causing all the thoughts?

Any of your thoughts with "I have to / should / need," "I am," or "s/he should/has/needs" or any other sentence that isn't objective. These sentences are thoughts we tell ourselves. Sometimes they're true and helpful while at other times they limit us.

Pick one of your thoughts to analyze closer. Doesn't matter which one. Just pick one that seems the most intriguing to you.

Read that thought out loud then answer these questions, in any order that feels right to you.

- What is your thought?
- What is the problem that you're having this thought about?
- How is having this thought helping you?
- How does saying that thought make you feel?
- When you say that thought or feel that emotion, how do you react?
- Is that thought true? Is it absolutely true?

This process is an effective way to analyze what thoughts and beliefs are holding you back and to create an awareness of your brain's dialogue. The best piece of advice when doing this work is to mainly focus on the thinking that's holding you back rather than only on the good ones. Those negative thought habits are golden nuggets that will help you find the health and freedom you're desiring.

Don't dismiss any thought that comes up. Typically, we toss out the first one that bubbles up. That first one, my friend, is usually your Inner Wisdom stating your truth before your primitive hindbrain overrides the thought.

Lastly, be honest with yourself as you do your brain dumps and thought analyses. Holding yourself to integrity is also a space for making adjustments aligned with your intentions.

This exercise is one of creating an awareness of what you're thinking. Doing a quick brain dump and analysis, even on a cocktail napkin, anytime you're feeling the weight of thought spirals or emotions will help you feel better and think intentionally. You're becoming conscious of the unconscious, which will help you to reset your health and life.

One moment I'm working on a project when suddenly the realization kicks in that I'm working on an unrelated task. Have you ever had that happen to you? Hyper-focusing is one of my superpowers, or so I thought. Even superpowers can discharge inefficiency. I suspect that my deep thinker tendencies contribute to being able to hyper focus. The unawareness of shifting tasks rattled me. One moment I was working on a blog and then next scrolling through Facebook. My body was humming, my heart racing, and my breathing practically stopped. This was my signal to pause, apply C.A.L.M.R., and do a brain dump to see what was going on. 15 minutes later I was back on track.

CLEANING UP AND RESHAPING THOUGHTS

Data collectors love to find patterns and categorize. Being trained in collecting data for behavior, I kept track of all thoughts and how often

I heard them. We all have our own personal playlist running in our brains. I encourage you to list any thought patterns that you discover.

Once you have found thoughts working against you the time has come to give them a bath and cleanse them! I used to think that I always had to be available in my job. I had convinced myself that I always had to cover for staff when they were ill or on vacation, staying alert to emails and requests, and always saying yes to projects and assignments. What if the "I always had to be available" mentality meant I worked within the parameters of my job? Then I would have created a coverage process rather than jumping in to do the work adding 20 extra hours to my week. No wonder I became exhausted!

Many high achievers think they haven't learned enough yet. That "I haven't learned enough yet" thought stops them from putting their knowledge to work. Instead, they're busy taking more classes, workshops, and courses. They're not giving themselves the time needed to become competent. The discomfort of feeling incompetent and the fear of failing are paralyzing. Their thought that "learning more is needed" is an error that's keeping them stuck. What if that high achiever thought that she "knows enough right now"? Well, she gains experience, uses mistakes and failures as feedback for growth, and considers further training as she's becoming unconsciously competent. She contributes as planned while gaining valuable experience.

Cleansing and reshaping unhelpful thoughts is easy in theory. First, you need to know what thoughts you consistently have. Check your list from your brain dumps and analyses to find patterns. Select a thought that's not serving you well and reshape it by changing it from an unintentional thought into one that's intentional and conscious.

Reshape your thinking by asking yourself the following questions:

- Do you want to change your result? Yes? What would you like to happen?
- What needs to be done to make what you want happen? List everything you need to do.
- What emotion motivates you to do everything on your list?
- What thoughts can you think of that create the feeling you want that helps you do the things on your list?

- Say this new thought out loud. Feel the emotion that follows. Let the emotion flow through your body. Repeat 3 to 6 times or until it feels settled into your body.
- Repeat the step above before you set out to do a specific task or any time throughout the day.
- Write this affirmation in your journal, daily calendar and post it wherever you see it frequently as a reminder.

Taking a huge leap from "I don't know enough yet" to "I know enough right now" might not work. We had to learn basic math before jumping into geometry, trigonometry, algebra, and calculus, right? Breaking down a new clean thought into smaller, more digestible bites eases the transition. For example, you can soften "I don't know enough yet" to "I'm considering I know enough right now" or "I'm figuring out I know enough right now."

The best way to know if you split a new intentional thought well enough is that when you say it, you can feel its rightness. Relax and take a few deep cleansing breaths. Now, say aloud your new intentional thought, "I know enough now," take another deep breath and say it again. Are you feeling it in your body? No? Keep breathing and repeating until you do. If you don't then reshape the thought. A thought that's right feels light and non-constrictive. Even better, if your body feels light with a twinge of vomit then you're right on the mark. I encourage you to push the envelope just a smidge when you're practicing cleansing and reshaping your thoughts. The more you think your newly reshaped thought, the stronger your brain rewires.

QUIETING YOUR INNER CRITIC

Inner Critics are stifling and at times paralyzing. Every time Alana wanted to offer suggestions, feedback on a project, or ask a question she heard a voice in her head telling her that no one wanted to hear from her. That voice in her head is one of her Inner Critics. She has several but they show up only when she's about to participate in a meeting, write a proposal, or offer her art for sale. Listening to her

Inner Critic was holding her back from potential promotions and earning extra money from her side gig.

Inner Critics are full of judgments that, in the end, are self-abusive. We don't tolerate nor do we often say to others what we allow our own brain to say to ourselves. You might think that you're stuck with that inside voice screaming at you, but you're not. Listening and accepting judgment from your Inner Critic ruins your mood, creates self-hatred, stops forward momentum, makes us worry what others think, what we do, how or what we say or don't say, and reruns events from the past. Most of all, being ruled by your Inner Critic fuels your chronic fatigue cycle.

There are several ways to combat your Inner Critic to take back your power. Know that you don't have to feed your trolls! One of my favorite ways of working with Inner Critics has an artistic and creative flair about it. In your journal identify who your Inner Critics are then create fun names for each one. For example, one of my Inner Critics is named Harried Harriet. Harried Harriet is my Inner Critic who tells me to work faster so I can get to the next thing. By rushing I'm ignoring the way I work best, which is methodical and thoughtful because I want to savor learning and creating. There's also Perfectionist Patty who loves to tell me that my work is incomplete. Patty keeps me working overtime and questioning the value of my work.

Once your list is done, the creative and most fun part begins. Set aside a 2-page spread in your journal or a blank piece of paper. Pull out your crayons, markers, colored pencils, and glitter glue — this is going to be fun! Grab a stack of magazines to clip out pictures that you can glue into your journal then draw or doodle on top. Using pictures from magazines, royalty free images from the internet, or using a marker, draw one of your Inner Critics any way you like onto one page of your journal spread or blank piece of paper. You don't need to get fancy or even have artistic flair, drawing a simple stick person will do!

Now that your Inner Critic is identified and drawn, take a few moments to think about this specific critic. Take 15-20 minutes to respond to the following prompts on the blank page next to your Inner Critic:

- When you tell me [list everything this Inner Critic tells you] it makes me feel [list exactly how you feel]
- Write a short paragraph or journal what listening to your Inner Critic cost you
- Explain how exposing your Inner Critic is a benefit that will help you move forward

INNER CRITIC SELF-DEFENSE

For some reason we think that our Inner Critic is our source of wisdom. It's drilled into us to listen to our brain and not our hearts or what we somehow know is best for us. The Inner Critic is actually you repeating words heard and held onto from the past. Essentially, we're giving our power away to a voice stuck in our head that keeps us stuck in fear. A powerful technique that I learned from Alex Howard to quiet your Inner Critics is to defend yourself. Talking back to your Inner Critic is an effective way to take back your power.

Some of my clients find that telling their Inner Critic to "fuck off" quiets down its voice. My apologies for using such a strong curse word, but there is something awfully powerful when you shout "fuck" at a voice tossing hurtful insults and judgments. If saying such a strong curse word is not for you, then consider saying, "how dare you speak to me like that" or "stop your trash talk" instead. For a more heart-centered approach to quieting your Inner Critic, try saying, "Yes, I hear you, but I want to do it this way" or "I really don't care what you think" or "Stop. You're making me feel bad about myself."

One of my Inner Critics is very much a bully. One night after an especially rough day my Inner Bully raised her voice loudly as I tried to fall asleep. Hearing my bully's voice made my stomach constrict and heart rate increase as I felt anxiety rising to my chest and throat. "Of course you can't say that," my bully said as if she was right next to me. "Shut the fuck up!" I said aloud. Again, my bully started to say, but in a softer tone, "Of course, you ..." as I immediately interrupted with a stern, "Fuck off!" One last time my bully attempted to share her opinion in a soft whisper as I beat her to the punch with, "Stop. Go away!"

It's been a long time since I've heard her voice. As I sensed my bully fading away, I visualized adult me holding tight to child me in support and compassion. Sometimes an aggressive response silences the determined Inner Critic more than the heart-centered approach. Neither way is right or wrong. Experiment to see what works best for you.

The most important thing to know about your Inner Critic is that you don't have to listen or attach to anything they say, unless you want to. It's your choice to listen or not. Inner Critics may never go away but you can quiet their harsh words. Don't forget to show the adult and child you some support, kindness, and compassion. After all, that's what you're both asking for. Having the courage to identify, name, and understand how your Inner Critic is keeping you small contributes to interrupting your chronic fatigue cycle.

A CLEANSED MIND

A cleansed mind is one that is virtually free from spinning, out of control thoughts, which are replaced by thought awareness and intentional thinking. I've already given you a couple of tools to begin taking control over unruly thinking and the pesky Inner Critic. A spinning and unintentionally thinking mind, along with any unbalanced behavior habits, is a perfect recipe for disconnection between your body and the present moment.

A cleansed mind is exactly what an overthinker is in dire need of. Overthinking is exhausting! The exhaustion of overthinking, along with dismissing any underlying emotions, was how I lived for a long time. My awareness of my overthinking habit happened when I decided to take a day off from my busy work to enjoy training my dogs and hanging out with friends. In fact, my overthinking brain ruined my day. My day of fun started out early, loading up the dogs and hitting the road at sunrise. On my way to our destination my work phone began pinging. Even though I told everyone I was offline for the day, I still picked it up to respond. I couldn't help myself! By the time I arrived at the workshop, I was angry with myself for not holding up my boundary as much as about the situation I got pulled into. At that time, I didn't know how to manage my mind. I thought the problem would resolve quickly, but half the day went by with texts and calls. I was so angry with myself and the issue that my Inner Critic screamed at me while I tried to have fun. The disruption interfered with my learning and socializing with friends. I sat in a corner with my head burrowed in my phone. I was far from present whenever it was my turn to work my dog. I was so distracted that feedback from the instructor couldn't be heard. I literally could not hear her words. Everyone kept their distance that I swear the instructor, my friends, and even the dogs could feel the cruel, critical voices clamoring in my head. I was clearly sucked into my inner voice vortex. Outwardly, I was being snippy toward others in the room and even telling the instructor, "I'm sorry but I can't even hear your feedback right now." This is what overthinking about a circumstance that you have no control over can do if you don't manage your mind.

When you become mindful of what thoughts your brain offers you, you are able to show up as the person you want to be. You take that necessary pause to find stillness and take deep breaths. You reshape and reselect thoughts instead of letting unruly, rude, and demeaning criticism fill your head.

A cleansed and clear mind, without doubt, brings about a sense of calm, focus, clarity, and peace. Knowing you can manage and choose and create intentional and helpful thoughts is satisfying and empowering. Too often we give our power away to circumstances, instead of managing our minds with curiosity and love. Stillness and mindfulness add strength to knowing that you can handle any problem dropped on your doorstep.

ns Ten ~

Cultivating Your Heart by Befriending Emotions

Having and feeling emotions is a dirty little secret that society tells us is wrong. We've become a cognitive-based population that prides itself on logic. The best part of being human is that we have emotions. Emotions invite connection to others, allow us to tap into creativity, and act as our personal navigation system. The heart (emotions) and the mind are meant to work together. Suppressing our emotions is like sweeping dirt under the carpet until a big bump can be seen. While we don't show bumps, suppressing emotions can lead to health issues. My pent up anxiety manifested into stomach pains as a child that then later expressed itself as IBS symptoms prior to succumbing to chronic fatigue. Emotions aren't anything to be afraid of. They're very much part of being human and serve us best when we listen to and befriend them.

If suppressing emotions was an honors level class, I got straight A's. I was so good at ignoring what I felt that I nibbled my nails down to nubs, kept myself overbusy between work and hobbies, ate a high carbohydrate diet, loved shopping sprees, and overindulged in cocktails and wine. My tipping point came after a culmination of many years of suppressed emotions from childhood and a variety of challenging life events. There wasn't one specific emotion or thing, just an accumulation of stuff I had never dealt with and not honoring who I am. Like most of us, I didn't know what to do with what I was feeling. The point where I knew I lost myself was when I felt a darkened thunderhead slowly maneuvering directly overhead. The rumblings of anxiety, anger, sadness, and shame began softly then gradually amplified, producing a deafening roar in my body and mind. There was pressure and darkness, at first slowly yet quite quickly building up all around and inside of me. I heard all criticism and arguing inside my head loud and clear. In between the judgments, the roar of thoughts came in and out so quickly that I couldn't make out a single word. My emotions were clearly telling me I needed to reset my navigation gear.

All those hidden emotions made my body feel as though it was being squeezed hard in a vice. My body wanted to crumble to the ground, checked out into a fetal position, hidden away under a thick, comfortable blanket. It wanted to hide in a locked closet, or run far, far away as my heart pounded and respiration rate increased. Heavy fatigue weighed on me yet as I tried to sleep or nap my body vibrated with restlessness. My body responded with fever, aches, chills, night sweats, and nightmares on a regular basis. Tightly packed emotions can make you cry, hide, scream, hit, or have a total meltdown, me included. I suppressed the discomfort of the moment further and further into my body because I didn't know how to deal with it until my heart screamed, "Stop now or I'll make you stop."

Imagine pushing those uncomfortable, hurtful and aching emotions into a secret hidden room. You push and squeeze them in with all your might, then slam the door and lock it tight. That secret emotion room fills up more and more each time you shove in more emotions. One day those hidden emotions start knocking on the door wanting to come out. When the call goes unanswered, they begin to push and push more until the door begins to budge. That's what happened to me.

Whenever that secret emotion room begins to bulge, the brain sends you a signal to do what you can to barricade the door. Instead of dealing with the emotions, most head to the pantry for a snack cake, chips and dip, or the fridge for ice cream or a few of *Mom's Munchie's Skinny Mint* cookies kept hidden for special occasions. Perhaps you head to the bar for a cocktail or glass or bottle of wine or two. Maybe your guilty numbing agent is shopping for things you really don't want or need or binging on Netflix when you could be getting things done. We all have a go-to numbing agent. What's yours?

You're making a best ditch effort to protect and heal a wounded heart by employing a numbing agent. Resisting the emotions is keeping you shackled to pain and discomfort. The famous psychologist, *Carl Jung,* is known to have said, "What you resist, not only persists, but also grows in size." Indeed, what you resist persists and grows in size in the form of emotional suffering and exacerbated chronic fatigue and disease. The payback in this case happens to be more guilt, embarrassment, and shame rather than actual healing and taking forward steps. By resisting the emotion bopping about the body, you're making it worse by pushing and numbing it away.

The body and mind work in partnership. Their communication is a two-way street. Whether the emotions from the body arose first or the speedy thinking is not known. In my opinion, I think that at times the body simply reacts to cues in the environment and the brain responds to the body's message. Likewise, the brain may be reacting to a cue and the body responds appropriately, just like the doe grazing in a meadow who senses a change in the environment. Based on her experiences and intuition, she decides whether a predator is approaching or she's safe. If the body and mind communicate in a reciprocal manner, then we can't heal if we don't feel our emotions.

Subtle cues in the environment, a similar situation, specific words or tones, a touch or lack of touch, unmet expectations, and wild inner storytelling can trigger a response from a past or current challenging life event.

No one is exempt from having challenging life events. They can appear as mundane as a simple move from one city to another or they can be as severe as the pressure felt in an unhealthy relationship when your partner threatens to commit suicide if you leave them.

Life principles to keep in mind that kick off cleansing your heart are: 1) You are only responsible for your thoughts, behavior, and actions, and no one else's, 2) Your reality is shaped by your experiences, memories, and beliefs, 3) Undefined and uncommunicated expectations cause emotional pain, and 4) Be selective with who you share your story with.

Only you are responsible for your thoughts, behavior, and action. You're also not responsible for the thoughts, behavior, and actions of another. This doesn't mean that someone won't hurt your feelings and vice versa. Feeling hurt by another's harsh words is okay, but what can you learn from those words? Barbed words flung at you are usually due to the other person's own scarcity thoughts. Perhaps you are a reflection of what they wish for. In return they project back to you their own sadness and frustration rather than making changes to their own lives and thinking. The light in you frightens them or makes them jealous. Many people believe that they are the way they are. That change can't be made. They were born poor, so they believe they have to live life poor. This is not true at all. There is plenty of evidence of people who dramatically changed their life circumstances for the better. Don't let these types of people dull your shine.

When someone complains about the number of hard-earned letters behind your name or your accomplishments then they're projecting onto you their jealousy about what you achieved. Realizing that person is wishful for what you've done creates compassion. You can feel compassion and empathy because they don't believe enough in themselves to make what they want happen instead of feeling embarrassed or ashamed of what YOU accomplished. There is always a way to achieve what you want, always, even if you have to take the long and windy route. My parents instilled in me that I can do and achieve whatever I want. I took (and still take) that belief and run with it. Even though one chapter in my life ended, it doesn't mean the next one will be lackluster. Momentarily, I allowed a few people to make me feel like an imposter but I've taken back my power now.

Your reality is shaped by your experiences, memories, and beliefs. The wonderful thing is that these aren't written in stone. You have the ability to create a new reality anytime you want by taking what you don't like, shining a light on it, and changing it to what you do want. When that thing you're doing no longer flutters your heart, you don't have to keep going. My illness began when I started feeling unhappy, bored, and felt like I was chugging along. Every day was déjà vu like the movie, *Groundhog Day*. Each day I was focused on all the bad stuff in the past and present. Bringing to the forefront what wasn't working and what I was craving led me to do things that made my heart sing. I began to focus on happy memories, achievements big and small, and future possibilities. I questioned my thinking and feeling by asking what I was craving, wrote about what that might look like, and asked myself what if I shifted gears.

Growing up my mother always said, "Treat others the way you wish to be treated." I stopped engaging in gossip, sarcasm, and comparing myself to others. Any comparison I did make came through the lens of inspiration instead of through lack. When I felt wronged, I questioned the problem and what I was making the problem mean about me. I began the slow waltz with my obliger, helper, and achiever ways. I learned to negotiate and override the poor advice from my jury of Inner Critics. Most importantly, I learned to cleanse my heart by riding my emotional waves. These changes required gradual yet major shifts but were worth the very bumpy ride at times. Aligning myself to what feels good to me, I have made that uphill walk a lot less steep with a lot less heartache.

Undefined and uncommunicated expectations are at the top of the list for creating emotional pain. We bring a lot of emotional pain to ourselves by having expectations of others. We expect loved ones and friends to know exactly what we need, when we need it, and to give it to us without asking. It's right up there with making someone else's opinion matter more than our own.

For more than half my marriage, I expected my wonderful husband to sit, talk, and watch movies with me in the evening. Every night I'd sit on the sofa next to him with the tv on, often with a book in hand. Without fail this handsome man would fall asleep. He'd miss all the good parts of the movie, show, or game. In the early years I'd toss pillows at him, poke and prod, and shout at him to wake up to no avail. Boy, I would get frustrated! It was boring watching a movie without someone and he was supposed to keep me company anyway.

Having the expectation that my husband, the professional napper, was responsible for entertaining me in the evenings only made me upset and feel like he didn't want to spend time with me. We both worked long hours but different schedules. He's an early bird and I'm a night owl. My creative time is late afternoon while his best energy time is bright and early morning. He pops up out of bed pre-dawn all chirpy, happy, and ready to play the music loud while a slow, easy morning as the sun passes the horizon with little talk is perfect for me.

My pestering him about napping affected our relationship. Once I realized I had this uncommunicated expectation, I changed my point of view. The man works damn hard and his evening napping habit actually gives me an opportunity to watch a show I enjoy (football and hockey is not my jam), read a good book, or work on a creative project. There's less tension and bickering. Exactly the way we like it.

These unpublished protocols we have for people may sound silly, but they really do cause us more emotional strife than necessary. It's easy to expect a loved one to know what we need, especially with having chronic fatigue or mold toxicity. We expect them to understand how our symptoms feel even when we look perfectly fine from the outside. We expect people to know the intricate details of our illness. We expect them to cook the right foods and stop offering us brownies or a cocktail every night then believe they're the ones responsible for sabotaging our gut problems. We expect them to rub our feet to ease the aches, run our Epsom salt bath with extra lavender and lit candles, or bring home flowers just to cheer us up. If you're doing this, stop it. Holding people accountable to an unpublished manual you have for them is only hurting you.

Be selective with whom you share your stories. There will always be people who don't believe in Chronic Fatigue Syndrome or mold toxicity. I've been told by medical professionals, friends, co-workers, and even acquaintances to get more sleep and take Sudafed and clean my house for the mold. Brené Brown in *Gifts of Imperfection* talks about sharing your story only with **a person worthy of hearing it.** Talking about your illness is a story worth being told to the right person. That right person is one who listens without judgment or sugar coating the problem. Share your vulnerability with a loved one or friend who says, "That sucks," "I'm right here, say more," or holds you tight while you let it all out. They don't need to say anything to make you feel better. That's your job to work on your thinking to change your feelings. But, having someone to help you bear witness to all those emotions is soothing, freeing, and healthy.

Seeking attention in order to capture a connection or to commiserate on your infliction is bound to backfire. Selectivity and education are your best bet to find the connection and empathy you're needing. Know exactly what you need then ask the right person. You'll make mistakes for certain but don't let that stop you. There is a group of loving, attentive, and caring people out there willing to support you. If they don't want to hear it, then you get to decide what you want to share and not make their resistance become part of your story.

When I first got sick with chronic fatigue and mold illness, many people who I thought were friends mostly told me to "get some rest" then dove into topics they felt most comfortable dealing with. My closest friends asked thoughtful questions to learn more rather than making assumptions, like black toxic mold is an allergy versus a true illness with neurological implications. The people in my innermost social circle asked to be educated and lent me their shoulder and ear when needed. I provided them with simple information spoken in layman's terms and offered articles and videos if they were interested in learning more. For me it's easy to get caught up in all the scientific jargon, so I spare my family and friends by making it super simple. The important piece is that I don't allow those who are disinterested to get me down. I now know in which ring of my social circle my friends, close friends, and acquaintances lie. It's just not worth the extra energy to fret over certain people.

Without doubt, I could take my toxic mold exposure diagnosis and make a big dramatic event out of it. I could blame many people and situations. Social media is a fantastic forum to release anger, frustration, and sadness to inflict blame to prove that I'm a victim of my circumstance. Victim mentality only keeps you focused on negative aspects rather than setting yourself up for success and healing. Negativity and the pity party for one keeps your nervous system humming away spending energy on a non-tangible event. The exposure happened and I can't prove exposure occurred in one singular space. What's the point of making a big deal out of exposing a possible culprit? In this case, the point would be to place unsubstantiated blame so that I "feel" better. To be honest, I wouldn't feel better at all and I'd still be stuck and very sick. Unresolved anger and frustration keep the fires burning. Accepting what it offers gives you the opportunity to heal, learn what is best for you, and find a path to move toward.

Cultivating your heart by befriending your emotions feels like peaceful and calm waters at sunrise or sunset. A light, energetic vibration in your body that feels weirdly alive yet comforting. So far, you've surrendered the tether of a perceived reality, expectations, victimhood, and comparison to take back your power through awareness, acceptance, selectivity, responsibility, thought cleansing, and emotional resiliency. Ahh, doesn't that feel much better?

Dealing with emotions was the clincher in my own healing journey. For way too long I resisted that anything was wrong. I had been through multiple therapists and so I thought that I was surely cured. The thing is that inner wounds never go away. They continue to bubble up every once in a while, which is perfectly normal. Tending to them as needed lessens the intensity and invites patience along with confidence so that you can handle the roughness as storms come rolling through. You know the storm is temporary and riding it out finds calm waters.

Tending to my inner wounds was uncomfortable but didn't last long. Bringing curiosity to the table makes the experience interesting and not intimidating. Oftentimes we're afraid of emotional pain, thinking that it will bring us back into the past, hurt us in some way (it already has, my dear), or do irreparable harm. The way to healing is through feeling emotions. Feeling is the way to healing the hurts from challenging life events and breaking your chronic fatigue cycle.

Ignoring emotions keeps you stuck and prevents healing or learning the necessity of emotional resilience.

HEART CLEANSE

Settling into the comfy recliner to catch a nap as fatigue wore heavy. Tucked under a soft fleece throw, two dogs snuggled in. One to the left and one on the lap keeping me well tucked in and toasty warm. Easing the recliner back to nearly flat, I closed my eyes and took several slow, full, and deep breaths. Thoughts that moment were silent. Earlier thought work settled them right down. The house was quiet albeit the occasional chatter of the birds at the feeder. The perfect napping scenario except my body felt wired. With every deep relaxed moment, I'd abruptly awake. My body vibrated and buzzed with each interrupted moment. At this point frustration usually steps in. I toss and turn for a while then get up to do something else. This time, however, I became curious about this sensation and decided to ride it to see where it took me.

Laying there I turned my attention to the sensations going on in my body. The sensations I felt are what I call anxiety. Anxiety feels differently for everyone. The way I feel anxiety, you may not. The sensations were vibrating fast and felt like tiny ping pong balls lightly bouncing off the inside walls of my chest. My stomach feels as if I'm on a roller coaster as it flies down the first steep dip. As my stomach constricted, I noticed a hardness that was warm. In my mind's eye I saw a big round orange ball that started bright then faded to grey then to the diffuse sunlight in the room. Relaxation and calmness replaced that anxious feeling that I napped for two hours straight with no interruptions. I have been able to successfully nap ever since I allowed myself to truly feel this emotion that wanted to be heard and finish its cycle of being digested and metabolized. From beginning to end was mere minutes, and I befriended that emotion.

At the time I thought I had done all the necessary work. A heavy veil of fatigue remained around my eyes. Every day I was doing my thought work, managing my mind, and thinking about emotions.

I practiced trying to feel my emotions but maybe I wasn't ready to experience this intense emotion until this very moment. I find that we are always where we are supposed to be. Giving myself permission to explore with objectivity what I was feeling released this emotional block that took my healing to a new level. I felt clearer, grounded, peaceful, and weirdly awake. The clarity of being truly awake when you've had severe fatigue and brain fog for a long time is indeed a new feeling. And one that I plan to keep!

Looking back at this breakthrough I can't help but wonder if I began the healing of an old challenging life event wound. There were many times I didn't feel safe while sleeping in my former marriage. Perhaps that's what needed to be heard and befriended. Applying my skill of stillness while watching and feeling the sensations moving about my body as if I were an outsider clearly allowed what was stored to move on. Our wounds don't just disappear and will poke their heads up every now and again just like the waves of the ocean. Some days the waves will be small and calm while other days they may fluctuate intensity, from medium to huge crashing waves. The more you allow yourself to feel the emotions come and go like the tide, regardless of the intensity, the more you will feel better equipped to handle them.

THE EMOTIONAL CLEANSE

Clearing away emotions is simple in concept. Basically, you sit back and feel all the sensations in your body without naming or making the rumblings, vibrations, tingles, zips, zaps, warmth, coolness, tightness or softness, colors, or shapes mean anything. They just are what they are. Become an observer rather than a participant. Watch your thoughts and emotions as if you were watching a movie. The more you allow your emotions the better you will feel emotionally and physically.

If you have suffered a significant trauma or find this process at all unsettling on your own, I recommend working with a therapist whom you feel most comfortable with. There are many modalities to help people suffering from PTSD, sexual assault, domestic violence, or other traumatic experiences find relief.

Begin emotional cleansing by addressing mild to moderate intense emotions first. Once you get the hang of feeling the sensations in your body then gradually move into the more challenging emotions.

To get started you'll want a private and comfortable space, a cozy blanket in case you get chilled or just want to snuggle, a pillow for your head or under your knees if you choose to lie down, a journal and a pen. This exercise will take 10 — 30 minutes.

Step 1: Prepare your private cocoon area.

Step 2: Settle into a supportive position. You may sit, stand, or lie down for this exercise. If you're sitting, be sure that your bottom is supported on a chair with feet firmly on the floor. You can sit in lotus position or legs stretched out in front of you for this, too. If you choose to stand, be sure that your feet are on firm footing. Know that you may sit down at any time. And, if you choose to lie down then be sure that you are comfortable with a pillow under your head or knees. This exercise is more effective if you close your eyes; however, the choice is yours to keep them open.

Step 3: Think about a situation that brings up an emotion for you. Envision the situation, recall the conversation, think about what you were thinking and feeling. Stay here until you feel sensations moving through your body.

Step 4: Get curious as the sensations move about your body. Where is it? Describe what it feels like. Is it hot, warm, cold, moving, stagnant, tingly, sharp, dull, loose, tight? Does it have a color or shape to it? Do the sensations move as you notice and acknowledge the sensations? Where do they go? Do they change? If yes, how do they change?

Step 5: Hang out and follow the sensations until they dissipate, dissolve, or you feel moved to end the session.

Step 6: Spend 3-5 minutes writing in your journal about the experience. What did the sensations feel like? Where were they? How did they move or not? What was the situation? What thoughts were coming up for you?

EMOTIONAL CLEANSING WITH MEDITATION

Meditation is widely used as a self-care modality. There is an abundance of scientific research that supports the benefits of a meditation practice such as calming the nervous system, clearer thinking, and relaxation.

Most people think that meditation consists of hours upon hours of sitting in lotus position. This is not true at all. Indeed, there are people that seek and build hours long meditation practices. We all have choices. If doing meditation longer than 20 or 30 minutes isn't your thing then that's okay. Aim to start with 10 to 15 minutes on a three to five times a week basis.

The first meditation to practice is one that teaches you to feel your body, The Body Scan. Getting into your body through meditation reconnects the mind to the body. A disjointed communication system heats up and wears out the nervous system and your energy. Meditation balances the mind + body connection that's working in harmony with your nervous system to refuel your energy.

The Body Scan is a simple meditation that you can do for 5 — 10 minutes on your own, with or without music. There is an abundance of body scan meditations on YouTube and many of the meditation apps, such as Insight Timer, Calm, and Headspace.

All you need to do a Body Scan meditation is a comfortable spot. You can sit, stand, or lie down. The body scan meditation is perfect to do as you wake in the morning and as you settle in for sleep. Feel free to play soft meditation music or enjoy a quiet room. Set a time for at least 5-10 minutes.

Step 1: Prepare your private cocoon area.

Step 2: Settle into a supportive position. You may sit, stand, or lie down for this exercise. If you're sitting, be sure that your bottom is supported on a chair with feet firmly on the floor. You can sit in lotus position or legs stretched out in front of you for this, too. If you choose to stand, be sure that your feet are on firm footing. Know that you may sit down at any time. And, if you choose lie down then be sure that you are comfortable with a pillow under your head or knees. This exercise is more effective if you close your eyes to reduce outside sensory input; however, the choice is yours to keep them open.

Step 3: Take 3-6 full deep breaths that fill your belly up to your chest. Inhale through your nose and exhale through your mouth.

Step 4: Turn your attention to each body part. Pause for several breaths to notice how that area feels. You can start at your head and work your way down to your feet. Or start at your feet and work your way up to your head. Take several moments to breathe into any tension to encourage relaxation.

Step 5: Take as much time as you want or need scanning your body. Notice any sensations. There is no need to name or make an interpretation of them.

Step 6: When you're ready, take your time coming back to the present moment. Notice how you feel now.

The Emotional Cleanse and Body Scan meditations are a great way to dip your toes into discovering that emotions aren't harmful. They're messages between the body and brain made by biochemical reactions within the body. The human body is equipped to process, digest, metabolize, and eliminate the metabolic waste of emotions, or we wouldn't have them. Fear of emotions causes stagnation that builds up until a trigger implodes the pile.

EMOTIONAL CLEANSE: EMOTIONAL FREEDOM TECHNIQUE

There came a point in my inner work that I still felt stuck. Shifting into my new identity, which is really about becoming me as myself, was hard work. Emotions and shadows from within needed to be spotlighted and coaxed out into the open. Tending my mind wasn't quite working as I recognized a pattern of inaction masked as busyness while I was building my coaching, daily self-care practices, and stepping out as the real me. My untended anxiety showed up as distraction, procrastination, and bouts of fatigue as I planned and prepared to take action in my new identity. This feeling was one I've felt most of my life but disregarded. I knew if I didn't address this constriction that I'd continue to swirl in stuckness. What I was feeling needed an oxy wash boost to release.

My biggest breakthrough came from an Emotional Freedom Technique (EFT), coaching session. I had great ideas about building my new career as a life and health coach yet struggled with expressing my identity, shifting it from who I was in the past to who I am now in the present moment. The funny thing is that my formal behavior education mostly focused on human behavior, which has set me up for everything I've done in my life including creating new chapters. It's really interesting where our brain and emotions go sometimes as we start stepping into something new.

My coach and I dove into my thoughts and feelings around who I was becoming to find the crux of what was holding me back. I was afraid of criticism and judgment from others, especially from my old career. I was hiding behind fear and shame. While we talked about my thoughts and feelings on this transition, my coach had me tap along meridian points (you'll learn more about those coming up). I basically gave a thought download and thinking cascade while gently tapping on points around my face, chest, ribs, and head. Fear and shame felt like constriction around my lungs and chest with a stuck sensation in the middle of my throat. Tapping along I likened the constriction to a fine bottle of champagne waiting to be enjoyed but the cork was too tight. Next thing I know the cork burst away as we tapped about what I could create with the fear and shame gone. Those emotions keeping me stuck popped out to let the sunshine bubble out! Peace and calm replaced the tension while ideas flowed like water.

Being coached through a situation with EFT is freeing and helps me take my power back at a higher level. To me this is what freedom feels like — calm, focused, peaceful, surety, trust. The tapping helped my body process the emotions while I talked about my situation. The emotional processing opened the door for what I wanted to feel as I stepped into the new me. Without that particular session, I doubt this book would be complete. I struggled writing, and it wasn't until this breakthrough session that the words began to flow. That's how powerful EFT is with taking back your power.

The world of Emotional Freedom Technique (EFT), otherwise known as "tapping," was introduced to me by one of my mentor coaches. EFT was originally developed by psychologist Dr. Roger Callahan in the 1980's, which was then called Thought Field Therapy (TFT). Gary Craig, one of Dr. Callahan's students further developed EFT. EFT is a gentle and highly effective technique for processing and releasing emotions, thoughts, and beliefs causing discomfort and stress. Tapping is a well-researched, scientific approach to releasing emotions by tapping with your fingertips on certain acupuncture meridian points while talking about your thoughts and feelings to unblock stuck energy.

Meridians are part of the body's energy system. Tapping on specific areas on the body's energy highway of meridians unclogs stuck energy, encourages energy flow, and delivers calming signals to the brain.

The efficacy of acupuncture is well documented, including EFT. As a tool, EFT is one that I use frequently with my coaching clients. It's simple and can be done most anywhere. You can say your thoughts aloud or in your head as you gently tap your fingers along the meridian points on your face, chest, and head.

The tapping points begin on the cushy area between your pinky and wrist, or what's called the "karate chop" point. The sequence after the karate chop point begins above your eyebrow closest to your nose.

Then move to the side of your eye, under your eye, under your nose, chin, along the collar bone, under the arm, then the top of your head.

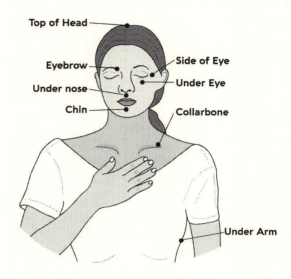

Figure 4: The EFT Tapping Points

Use your fingers or tap the cushy area between your pinky and wrist together while you say out loud or to yourself, "Even though I have [anxiety/sadness/fear/overwhelm], I deeply and completely accept myself." Say this sentence three times.

After saying your set-up statement while tapping on your karate chop points, move on to tapping each sequential tapping point, firmly yet gently 7-10 times. Say out loud or silently in your head about how you feel, what you think, and how you react as you tap along each meridian point.

Do a couple of rounds then pause to check in with how you're feeling. Begin again if you wish. Be patient with this process. There are times a block is immediately removed. Other times it may take a few hours, days, weeks, or more for results to reveal themselves. No change usually means there's more underneath to unravel.

At any time you wish to reduce stress and anxiety to encourage relaxation, tap on the meridians while focusing on your breath. It's okay to omit tapping on your karate chop points if you're tapping and breathing. Tapping as you slip under the covers for the night, stuck in traffic, or feeling an emotion rising is easy, effective, and a technique you can do yourself.

ACTIVITIES SUPPORTING THE EMOTIONAL CLEANSE

The first day at the work site was full of one problem after the next. Every attempt at problem solving led to dead ends in an endless maze of unhappy people, broken technology, and an upsetting incident that could have been prevented. Arriving at the site mentally and physically exhausted from the previous weeklong assignment with barely any down time in between, my stack of emotions began to teeter. One final demand tripped the trigger then the inner rumblings began. The urge to throw the computer, cell phone, and verbally lash out at anyone nearby was mighty strong. Instead of reacting to the rising tantrum, the cell phone remained on the table as I headed out the door for fresh air and a walk to calm myself.

Once back at the hotel I changed into workout clothes, grabbed my headset and iPhone, and headed down to the hotel gym, where I hopped on the treadmill with my favorite tunes blasting in my ears. I set my pace to match the intensity of the anger and frustration I felt about the day. I allowed my feelings to move my body to the beat of music and watched my thoughts fly by. I let them all go by focusing on the pace and intensity of my speed walk. About two miles in I was able to decrease the intensity of my pace. An hour later, I stepped off the treadmill ready to clean up and grab a bite to eat.

Because we aren't taught how to deal with emotions, we often allow them to run us. There's a choice we have of whether to chuck that cell phone against a wall or the floor while screaming obscenities or to simply walk away, ride the emotional wave, then make a plan when the waters calm down.

There are a multitude of ways that assist emotional processing without exploding like a bomb.

Movement is one of the best ways to get your emotions moving along. Daily walks or runs. For those who haven't been able to exercise, begin taking short walks from the bedroom to the living room, down the driveway, part way down the street, then around the block.

Dancing around the house or joining a dance class is a fun way to get movement in along with connection with your partner. Slowly moving your body to your favorite song is movement. Dance, sway, tap your toes, and gracefully move your arms to the rhythm. Who cares if you got the right moves or not? What matters is that you find movement you enjoy.

Yoga and Pilates are gentle ways to move your body while connecting to your breath. There are different types of yoga and Pilates. Investigate the differences and try out the ones that interest you. Some classes use props. Some can be more vigorous while others are more gentle.

The options are numerous. Select ones that you enjoy. For me I regularly go on hikes in the woods with my dogs because I love being outdoors and in nature, attend Pilates and yoga classes, and ballroom dance with my main man. We love dancing East Coast Swing, Fox Trot, Rumba, and Cha Cha, which is the perfect date night activity for fun and connection.

Breathwork helps release emotions like anxiety, grief, and anger trapped in our body. Breathwork is also called pranayama. According to James Nestor, author of *Breathe*, humans have evolved to have smaller and more narrow mouths. This means our breathing is shallow and takes in less oxygen, which affects our sleep, body function, and healing. Our bodies run on not only nutritious food but on oxygen. Breathwork not only moves along emotions but energizes and feeds your nervous system.

Many yoga classes include short pranayama exercises in their sessions. A simple breath pattern for relaxation is the 4 Square Breath Pattern. Inhale through the nose to a count of 4, hold breath for 4, exhale through your mouth for 4, hold for 4 then start the cycle again.

There are more vigorous breath patterns that move emotions effectively. My favorite is the Tri-Active breath pattern. In this breath pattern you inhale twice filling your belly then chest and exhaling with an audible sigh. Continue this breath pattern for 10-30 minutes. Be aware to set a comfortable pace and maintain deep inhales to the breath pattern. Fast or shallow breath inhalations can lead to tetany. Tetany is when your hands cramp up into a claw shape due to a lack of oxygen input. You will want to lay down on the floor on a yoga mat. Place a bolster under your knees. Have a comfy blanket nearby because you're likely to get chilled with breathwork. Notice the sensations but refrain from naming or interpreting them. Journaling after a breathwork session offers great insight. Emotional release from breathwork offers clarity, relaxation, and focus.

Nature is one of the most serene and healing places to be. No matter where you live, step into the outdoors. The fresh air, plants, streams, mini waterfalls, ponds, lakes, and oceans, birds singing and flitting about, and wildlife, be it squirrels or chipmunks, have a wonderful effect on our body and mind. In our current times, human life is mostly focused on the indoors with the invention of air conditioning and heating systems and office work instead of farm work. We're not as connected to the ecosystem as our earlier generation. Take a walk in the park, hug a tree or at least sit under one, or take a stroll on the beach or ride a bike on a trail. Use all your senses on your walk about, ride, or sit down. Feel the breeze, smell the ocean air or fresh cut grass, hear the birds, and drink in the details of a flower. Drink in this elixir of life.

Journaling is not only a place to write down your thoughts. Give yourself permission to write about your emotional experiences. A regular journaling practice helps keep rogue emotions in check and offers an outlet. This is a place not just to analyze thinking patterns keeping you stuck. Journaling is an opportunity to get honest with yourself about what you're thinking and feeling.

Art Journaling is a practice of drawing and writing about your emotions. Write out your feelings then cover them with a variety of paints, pictures, stamps, quotes, drawings, colors, and textures. Art journaling engages the right side of the brain, the creative and intuitive side. The left brain is analytical and logical. Engaging your right brain invites thought and emotional processing. Plus, it's so much fun!

Singing is another way to get those emotions out. Sing to your heart's content with your favorite song. Remember when you were a kid and would sing into your hairbrush in the mirror because you knew you'd be a rock star? Step back in time when you were alone in your bedroom singing along with your favorite rock star using a hairbrush as the microphone. Allow yourself to sing at the top of your lungs in the shower, kitchen, when you're driving around town, or wherever!

Laughter, especially a gut-busting laugh, makes anyone feel better. Think about what makes you laugh the most and seek it out. Recall conversations with your best girlfriends where you all almost peed your pants or blew wine out your noses. How did you feel after those times? Amazing, right? Laughter helps get those emotions processed, digested, and metabolized.

Play is an ingredient to finding your sweet spot. When you're at play, say art journaling or scrapbooking or knitting, the time flies by. What seems to be 20 minutes has actually been 2 hours. This is play. Play can be any fun and playful interaction with your spouse, children, friends, pets, or on your own. What is playful for you?

The above tools and tips are things to incorporate into your daily routine to help keep your physical and emotional body balanced. You might like a structured approach or prefer free form. Either way, they take up as much time as you dedicate and can be used in a pinch. Decide and try on different ways to add these activities into your daily routine.

Emotional cleansing is about living *in* your life, not just living life, including taking in and embracing human experiences within and outside of you. Living life is like an unmoored ship in the open ocean meandering along every current without a plan or strategy to steer in the right direction when the storms come rushing in. An unmanned ship gets battered with a high risk of tipping and sinking to the bottom where it lays in perpetual rest.

Living *in* your life is about that easy cruise in the Caribbean with warm tropical breezes and frequent stops to investigate the ocean's coral reefs by snorkeling or scuba diving. It is about slow swims in the turquoise blue, warm waters, and lounging on deck taking in the beautiful sights of the islands. Tranquility and peace fill most days even though the threat of storms and hurricanes occasionally make an appearance. The change in the air, clouds, and winds are cues triggering activation of storm proofing by battening down the hatches and collecting supplies to ride out the apparent incoming storm. Tools and skills are at hand to handle any crisis that arises.

The unpredictability of the ocean reflects the unpredictability of human life. Storms roll across the ocean periodically as they do for you and me. If we were only to experience happiness, then what would sadness mean? The spectrum of emotions is part of the human experience. Our job is to figure out how to ride the occasional storms in a way that not only protects us but catapults us in the right direction by experiencing our emotions and managing our minds around those experiences.

While writing this book I learned that toxic mold still resided in my body after a year of treatment with the prospect of yet another year of treatment ahead of me. All sorts of emotions ran through me. Anger that I was exposed, that my voice wasn't heard, and that we never noticed mold silently growing in our basement. Grief ran through me, grief that I wasted too much time and should have sought help sooner. Frustration showed up for not being where I wanted to be. Using the tools described above helped me ride out the storm of emotions brewing inside. I had already done a lot of emotional cleansing work so this time around they needed a wipe down rather than a full cleansing.

Feeling the anger, grief, and frustration allowed the emotions to move. There was no wallowing or ruminating. I let those feelings have their say. Afterward I turned my focus toward gratitude, toward what is next. Gratitude that mold helped me see and shine my own light, taught me how to truly slow down, and to discover the me who wanted to be found. Gratitude that I know how to tweak and adjust the plan to escort remaining mycotoxins trying to cling on. Excitement joins gratitude that more energy is on the way as I continue pushing mycotoxins out, minding my mind, befriending emotions, and tending to my soul.

When you cultivate your heart by befriending your emotions the nervous system settles down and moves back toward homeostasis.

There's space to breathe with a sense of ease and peace within. Doing the inner work of emotional cleansing was my major breakthrough that got me unstuck in my healing process. Becoming curious and having the willingness to explore my emotions repaired many energy leaks from within. My work is not done because these leaks will require maintenance from time to time. But now I have the tools and skill to direct my energy in more purposeful ways.

Eleven

Cultivating Your Soul Through Self Advocacy

Old habits die hard. In the early months and years of my healing journey I'd find myself repeating habits that depleted a lot of energy. The feeling of missing out was a big one. Achiever, helper, and obliger tendencies kept me on the competition trail when I needed to slow down and do a lot less. The idea of missing out on winning a class, earning a qualifier or a podium appearance, disappointing my husband, and missing out on connecting with friends was still strong. The playful joy of running a course with my dogs was an addiction that I made into work rather than play. The stress of early morning starts, juggling three dogs, and being sensitive to the lights and noise were too much for my body. I gave myself plenty of time to recover during the week but every weekend the warrior came out to push through another two or three days of competition, travel, and socialization.

The imbalance of my achiever, helper, and obliger ways interfered with the joy I once had at competitions. The very thought of preparing for a weekend away sent my mind into a flurry of getting it all done then worrying about having enough energy to unpack only to do it all over again the next week. The thought that saying no wasn't available to me kept me spinning in overwhelm. I was exhausted even before I arrived.

Most of the time I didn't allow myself to even feel the pride and joy of success. Perfection doesn't exist and there's always more to fix and improve upon. The most interesting thing of all is that this pattern is how I've handled most areas of my life. I'd push and drive to succeed then celebrate with a dose of self-criticism that what I accomplished wasn't good enough or I should've said no to the invite.

Imbalanced behavior and thinking habits contribute heavily to internal stress. That stress keeps the nervous system running at full tilt, gobbling up precious fuel that could be allocated to healing your body.

Self-advocacy is about taking back your power by taking care of and being responsible for your own needs. You've always had your power. It's just that your ruby shoes slipped off. Taking back your power relies on you putting back on the sparkly ruby red shoes and tending to your mind, heart, and soul. It's time to treat yourself like you wish to be treated. Become an energy strategist by designing a life you rightfully deserve with solid boundaries protecting your precious energy, putting the oxygen mask on yourself as an act of self-love, designing experiences you want to have, and creating a soul tending basket in preparation for the rough days.

BOUNDARIES

Being eager to please others, the answer was always yes. The answer was yes to prove you're a team player. You want to show you have value, knowledge, and skills, but you also don't want to miss out on any of the action. You frequently check texts and emails throughout the day and night, even when you're on that hot date with your husband or are celebrating the holidays with your family. That eagerness interferes with being present with the ones you love most, including yourself. Such eagerness is selling your soul to the devil because soon they'll figure out that you're always available. Then the day that you truly aren't available an argument ensues because you're *always* available. Do you give up your plan or figure out how to squeeze in the request when you're supposed to be somewhere else to make the requester happy? There's no doubt that the persistent requesters will track you down no matter where you are, even if you're in the middle of the bush in Africa or hidden away in a wood burning sauna in a refurbished Swedish mill house with poor cell reception. Requesters become like annoying mosquitos buzzing around trying to land to get a sip of your precious energy.

For the one who's always available, an internal struggle ensues. Because a boundary wasn't made in the early stages, the consequence becomes do it or be reprimanded while anger, anxiety, and frustration brew inside forcing you outside a healing state. This is the stage that obligers and helpers set when they're too willing to say yes.

The idea that boundaries are for others is a misconception. Boundaries are for *you*. Boundaries aren't ultimatums or handed out indiscriminately. Boundaries help you balance out your behavior habit tendencies.

A great boundary to create if you're an obliger or helper type is to tell the requestor that you need to check your schedule and will get back to them with an answer by [insert day/time]. This gives you the opportunity to take a few moments to check your calendar and ask yourself if you truly want to take on the request.

At first the requester may be taken off guard, especially if in the past you've always immediately said yes. This is okay because it's a start. Their thoughts and interpretations about why you need to get back to them is on them, not you. Each time you respond this way then the requester figures out that you need extra time and willingly offers it or finds someone else. The bottom line is that everyone is out for themselves. Follow the lead and start advocating for you.

Many achievers like to have a lot of activities on their plate. Installing a boundary, such as only taking one online course at a time, eases the pressure achievers put on themselves. Limiting the number of activities offers the opportunity to focus and absorb the information you're learning while overwhelm dissipates.

Maybe you're trying to rest but are consistently interrupted by children, spouses, or the notification pings on your phone. A boundary you may need to set is that when you're resting, you will ignore all requests unless there's blood or death involved, at least until you emerge. At that time, you will answer questions, play, make a snack, etc. Now, you need to consider a consequence if your boundary is broken. A consequence could be that you will lock the door and not respond unless there is blood or death. You get to decide. It's key to lay out the boundary clearly to the requester before activating your boundary. It's not fair and is an expectation that will cause you more stress by setting yourself up for anger and frustration if you don't clearly outline the rule.

One boundary I wished that I communicated was around office hours. My overexuberant obliger tendencies had me tied to my phone and responding at all hours. By the time I understood how boundaries worked (clearly defining and communicating them) I already had people well trained to know that I was always available. Setting a boundary around office hours was the best thing despite the challenge of implementation. The struggle was real on everyone's part but with perseverance and consistency the boundary stuck.

Creating boundaries is a powerful skill that fills the energy tank. Boundaries are the ultimate in self-care. The only obligation you have is to you, unless you decide to commit to an activity, task, or responsibility. Even then, boundaries are available to save you from energy depletion so you can then give from a cup that is full or overfull rather than half full.

POWER OF SELF-LOVE

Staring at the calendar against the list of projects, trips, activities, and to-do's, the sense of deep overwhelm built up from the stomach upwards. Thoughts whirled at a high rate of speed while trying to organize the list of priorities made everything unclear. The pressure from the outside, although perceived, caused snarky responses to others and within my mind. Oh, my Inner Critics had a field day. The inability to ask for help set a belief that only I could get the items done correctly. No delegation or asking for help are allowed. As a result, I spun in the overwhelm with an impossibly long to-do list. The jury of Inner Critics shouted loudly that nothing will get done, I'm doing it wrong, and am a failure for not managing properly.

The need to do it all brought along feelings of inadequacy, doubt, and no self-worth. Feeling that my to-do list was my responsibility, I was consistently failing to complete every task on my overfull list. This failure projected itself as worthlessness on my part. In the end, I accepted the harsh verdict of my Inner Critics.

Our jury of critics is all too happy to dish out harsh criticism and we're all too happy to accept it. Self-love simmers down the abuse Inner Critics dish out. Accepting and believing the gaslighting our Inner Critics spout out is an abusive environment. You have the choice to continue living in that environment or not. A way out is through self-love.

Self-love is accepting and honoring your value and enough-ness as you are. Self-love spotlights all your goodness, talents, skills and encourages you to the heart. Self-love is accepting all of you as you are even those cute little quirks. Self-love is your BFF who's got your back, reminds you to shine your light bright, and cheerleads the way. We're all unique, which makes us all special in a wonderful way. How boring would it be if we were all perfectly alike? Self-love is treating yourself the way you treat others with love, offering your body food that fuels, giving yourself a compassionate hug, and speaking to yourself in a kind and supportive manner.

Self-love is not selfish. Not even one iota of selfishness is in self-love. How can you give love if you don't love you? Loving yourself first opens the door to loving at a higher level, the way you want to love because you know that you're loved and there's lots of love to give.

When you love who you are then you show up as the loving person you are. Knowing you've got your own back through body, mind, heart, and soul tending, you can love with your whole heart. Not a quarter or half heart, but a full heart and more. Here are four activities to begin loving you:

1. **I See You** is a great place to start seeing you. Take a good hard look at yourself in the mirror. Look at her straight in the eye. Hold your eye contact. Look at her. What do you see? What are all the good things that you see? What does she have to say? Give her the honor of listening. Then spend a little time writing down what she had to say in your journal. These are gold nuggets to work on and grow from.

2. **Morning Reconnection** is a great way to wake up in the morning. The process is simple and as luxurious as you want. As you awaken, lay still and do a body scan while taking slow, deep breaths. Stay here a while then when ready, ask yourself what do I need today? Continue breathing and an answer should come. If not, keep trying, especially if this kind of process is new to you.

3. **Love Spots** are reminders to yourself about all your awesomeness. Place them where they can be seen easily. Say them out loud. Let the words reverberate into your body. Keep a list handy to refer to whenever you need an extra boost of how valuable, worthy, and enough you are.

4. **Self-Love Letters** are in-depth reminders of all the wonderfulness of you. Write yourself a Love Letter describing all the positive aspects of who you truly are. Be honest and tell your Inner Critics that they've already had their say and now it's your turn. Tuck this letter away to read any time your spirit needs to be lifted.

Tiny daily acts of self-love boosts self-worth. Your morning, afternoon or evening practice of meditation, self reflection, movement, and play are acts of self-love. Self-love invites confidence as you design a life that supports your healing and recovery needs. You are worth every single drop.

DESIGN YOUR EXPERIENCES

Just the thought of stepping back into the ring with my dog by my side led to a slew of negative thought loops. The "I have to go," "I have to run in every class," "I won't get quality sleep," and "this is what I do" thoughts build a lot of stress. That stress turns into a sense of dread and pressure to play a sport I love with my dogs. This same pattern ran through my mind about all my work travels, too. It's fascinating how stuck we get in patterns.

Inner work offers freedom to choose what you want to feel and experience. Thus, interrupting and redirecting old patterns to enjoy events and experiences are in your control.

Dig deep into your thoughts and feelings about certain events like visits with a loved one, work, or an activity you engage in. Examine why you enjoy and dislike the activity. Do you want to continue the activity? Why or why not? If you decide that you want to continue the activity, what would you like to experience? How would you feel? Are there thoughts that can be adjusted to help you feel the way you want?

The fretting and stress stopped when I explored why competitions were becoming stressful for me. Deep down I didn't want to quit. I took time to think about how I want to experience competitions. Then I set about creating that experience reminding myself what I want to experience and focusing on thoughts that bring the feeling I want to have. I prepare the day before by visualizing the entire day from waking up to settling into bed for the night.

When my experience shifted significantly toward the negative, I used this same technique around my work travels. Visualizing and creating the experience I wanted helped me to show up as the approachable professional leader that I am. I wanted to be present for all and create an environment that was supportive, creative, and collaborative. Staying focused on the negatives kept me in a space that created impatience, woeful thinking, and avoidance.

Envision what you want to experience in life, work, and play. Be specific about those experiences then start creating them step by step. There's no giant leap that will magically make everything change the next day. Begin by writing your specific vision as detailed as possible. Set boundaries. Take care of your emotional needs. Mind your mind. Nourish your body, mind, and heart. Bit by bit that vision will come true.

Competitions became my playground again. Selectivity and constraint in the amount of days and classes I participate in make a world of difference. An exciting side effect is that my dogs and I began to have more success with podium placements at large Regional and National events. My vision of a relaxed, playful, yet competitive experience strengthened my relationship with my dogs, husband, friends, and most importantly, me.

Traveling became fun again. Sharing knowledge, skills, and coaching other professionals was my sweet spot. Travel time became my nourishment time. Time to relax on the plane to immerse myself in a good book. Evenings in my hotel room became my sanctuary with aromatherapy, music, yoga, a good book, and time to practice my drawing skills.

This major shift in how I now interact in my chosen environments — personally and professionally — never would have happened without practicing self-love, managing my mind, and tending to my heart.

SOUL TENDING BASKET PREP

Focused on the computer screen you suddenly notice that Facebook is scrolling by instead of that document that needs to be written. Everything feels like it's moving through thick mud. Fatigue starts in the head slowly oozing down to the feet. You know what's next. A crash sending you to bed for hours or days.

Frantically, your mind starts telling you exactly how you got yourself to this point. The mind loves to tell you about all the work that will pile up while adding more fuel to the fire. You feel overrun, disappointed, frustrated, and just want to get on with life.

Take note of the signals notifying you that it's time to slow down. It's a message from your body asking for a little help. Morning Reconnection time is helpful to checking in with your body, to hear what it needs. This is the time to listen and start tending and not time to give yourself a shake down.

One of my mentor coaches inspired me to create a first aid kit to help nourish my mind, body, and heart when my body needs a rest. Being creative, I had a lot of fun building my first aid kit, which I now call a Care Tending Basket. I invite you to build your own basket or box or bag any way you want.

My Care Tending Basket holds reminders, inspiration, books, and paper. The basket is placed where I can see it to remind me of its purpose. Opening the basket, I will find affirmations written on pretty cards, reminders of what I enjoy like tea, Epsom salt baths, and a nap under a cozy warm blanket. Essential oils that calm and soothe are ready to dab onto points on my wrists, neck, and face. One of my cards lists movies that lift my spirit and a note to head to the meditative spa channel on Pandora to soothe the nerves. Reminders that slowing down makes things happen and I'm exactly where I need to be to keep me on track despite the interruption. Several small inspirational books written by Maya Angelo, Mister Rogers, and Janet Archer beckon to be read. A sketch and note pad, pack of crayons, graphite pencils, and a good old Bic pen invite me to write, draw, and color to get out of my head and into my heart. I get to pick and choose depending on what strikes my attention. I might write, draw, read, meditate, take a hot bath with a good book, or take a nap with my cozy throw and a dog or two keeping me warm.

The push-through mentality encourages dismissing the signals our bodies send. Check in to determine what type of tired you are. Have you been doing a lot of thinking or mentally intensive work? Taking a break to go for a quick walk might be more worthwhile than an hour's nap. Did you just experience an intense emotional event? Tending to your heart is the next step. Or is your body telling you that it truly needs a break? Make a selection or two that speaks to you from your Care Tending Basket that will nourish your body, mind, heart and soul. These acts are self-love and compassion.

To create your own basket, select a special box, bag, or basket that will hold your soul tending ideas, reminders, book, and journal.

Choose items that make you feel inspired. Slip a packet or two of your favorite tea, a favorite essential oil scent, a candle, a note to call a supportive friend, or a list of movies. When you're done, set your Soul Tending Basket where it's easily accessible. Place your basket where you see it to serve as a reminder that help isn't far away.

Care tending is at the heart of tending your soul. Self-care is soul tending. Tending to your body, mind, heart, and soul leads to healing and energy creation.

Conclusion

The Gift of Chronic Fatigue

Recovering from any illness or serious injury is a journey. It's a journey filled with a lot of bushwhacking, steep uphill climbs, followed by easy hiking through flat terrain before another steep uphill climb with a huge boulder blocking the way. Navigating the boulder is the way to find the next path as you climb the mountain called recovery. Some will discover a full recovery while others will be able to keep most symptoms at bay. Healing is a journey that's as individual as you. You have the choice to take what you will from your illness.

Chronic fatigue helped me find time for myself, time I lost in the craziness of the world and life. Chronic fatigue opened the doors to my superpowers and taught me to lean into my inner wisdom to shine brightly, to heal old wounds, speak up, and be seen.

The gratitude I hold for the message toxic mold had for me is immense. Toxic mold taught me to stop then slow down, search for and heal my inside world, align to what feels good to me, step out from hiding, let the true me sparkle and shine, and let my voice ring as loud as this thoughtful, gentle soul wishes.

What are you making your chronic fatigue, autoimmune disease, or exposure to toxic mold mean about you? Acknowledge then let that old negative story go. Focus your attention on creating a new story that reflects the gifts of chronic fatigue and your uncorked beautiful version of you.

That constant feeling of restriction in my chest and throat is a bottle of French champagne ready to be released, savored, and celebrated. Within that constriction resides the effervescence of you and me. The bottle itself represents old wounds in hiding wanting to release their voices to finally be heard. Letting each voice speak in their own time invites the vice grip of chronic fatigue to release. It is your job to hear and feel them out.

The great psychologist Carl Jung said, *"Until you make the unconscious conscious, it will direct your life and you will call it fate."* For me, doing this inner work created a breakthrough that popped that champagne cork to let my effervescence of sparkle and shine burst through. Energy, clarity, and a sense of peace washed over my body. That sense of peace finally feels like it's come home.

My wish for you is that you explore the ideas I laid forth so that you, too, can find liberation by breaking your chronic fatigue cycle to create your best life on your terms. Release your heart-centered rebel because you are not broken, you are worthy, you are important, and you matter.

xo, Sharon

Review Inquiry

Hey, it's Sharon here.

I hope you've enjoyed the book, finding it both useful and fun. I have a favor to ask you.

Would you consider giving it a rating wherever you bought the book? Online book stores are more likely to promote a book when they feel good about its content, and reader reviews are a great barometer for a book's quality.

So please go to the website of wherever you bought the book, search for my name and the book title, and leave a review. If able, perhaps consider adding a picture of you holding the book. That increases the likelihood your review will be accepted!

Many thanks in advance,
Sharon Wirant

Will You Share the Love?

GET THIS BOOK FOR A FRIEND, ASSOCIATE OR FAMILY MEMBER!

If you have found this book valuable and know others who would find it useful, consider buying them a copy as a gift. Special bulk discounts are available if you would like your whole team or organization to benefit from reading this. Just contact hello@sharonwirant.com.

Would You Like Sharon to Speak to Your Organization?

BOOK SHARON WIRANT NOW!

Sharon accepts a limited number of speaking/coaching/training engagements each year. To learn how you can bring her message to your organization, call or email hello@sharonwirant.com.

About the Author

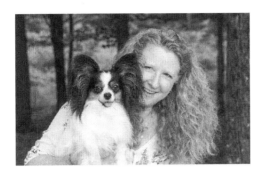

Sharon Wirant, MA is a behaviorist turned integrative coach who has a lifelong love for learning about personal development, self-care, and how all species engage with their environment. Sharon worked in the dynamic world of animal welfare for 20 years.

She discovered coaching when she struggled to understand why she felt so tired, stuck, and unfulfilled prior to her diagnosis of mono, adrenal fatigue, Lyme disease, and toxic mold illness. Unexpectedly, Sharon discovered that chronic fatigue is about more than a viral or toxin overload.

Sharon is known to be an avid researcher, outside-the-box thinker, and leader in her own quiet and thoughtful way. Inspired by her own recovery story, Sharon combines three unique skills to help others break their chronic fatigue cycle: personal development (life and health coaching), habit change (behavior and therapeutic coaching), and perseverance.

She shares her life with her husband, six dogs, a small flock of sheep, and a stealthy barn cat in beautiful New Hampshire.

Website: www.sharonwirant.com

Made in the USA
Middletown, DE
12 February 2023

24552676R00106